BODYTONING

CHRISTOPHER M. NORRIS

A&C Black • London

First published 2003 by A&C Black Publishers Ltd
37 Soho Square, London W1D 3QZ
www.acblack.com

ISBN 0 7136 6172 0

A CIP catalogue record for this book is available from the British Library.

Note: Whilst every effort has been made to ensure that the content of this book is as technically accurate and as sound as possible, neither the author nor the publisher can accept responsibility for any injury or loss sustained as a result of the use of this material.

Acknowledgements
Cover photography © ImageState
Illustrations by Jean Ashley
Photography by Grant Pritchard
Models: Stephen Aspinall, Stephen Bennett, Joanne Dawes, Anthony Greenhouse, Edwin Walsh.
Thanks to David Hammond and everyone at David Lloyd, Trafford Park, Manchester.
Designed and typeset by Fakenham Photosetting, Norfolk

A&C Black uses paper produced with elemental chlorine-free pulp, harvested from managed sustainable forests.

Printed in Singapore by Tien Wah Press (Pte.) Ltd.

DEDICATION ❮

For Hildegard and Sophie, my girls

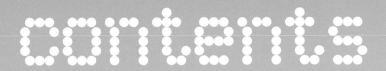

contents

BODYTONING
THE SCIENCE OF GYM BASED EXERCISE

BODYTONING FOR A BETTER LIFE

Our modern day lifestyle is considerably less active than that of our parents and grand-parents. Although the change from the heavy industry and 'hard graft' of the industrial revolution has brought with it many health benefits, it has also brought with it modern day health problems. Many of the infectious diseases of the last century have gone, to be replaced by heart and circulatory disorders as the number one cause of death. Exercise as part of a general lifestyle change is one of the most important factors in the prevention of these modern health problems. Equally, four out of five people suffer from severe back pain at some times in their lives, and this condition recurs in a staggering 60 per cent of cases. Again, exercise has been shown to be of overriding importance in both the prevention and treatment of this condition. The message is clear, *if you want to stay healthy, exercise regularly*.

In this book we will look at the safest and most effective ways to exercise using gym-based equipment. The principles and programmes are based on science rather than hearsay, an approach which takes away the guesswork involved in exercise selection.

Chapter 1 looks at the preparation for training and deals with the all important principles of warm-up. In chapters 2, 3 and 4 we will look at the way the body works and how exercise affects you when you work out. We then move on to exercise techniques and apparatus in chapters 5 and 6. For the practical side of the book, we will look at core stability, stretching and cardiovascular (CV) training to begin with and then move on to weight training using both machines and barbells and dumb-bells ('free weights'). We include non-weight exercises in the form of bands and stability balls, and then describe programmes for both fitness and to target the aches and pains which so often accompany a modern day lifestyle. Finishing with advanced techniques for sport, *Bodytoning* represents the complete guide to gym-based exercise.

WARM-UP

In terms of injury, the preparation we do before starting a workout can be more important than the contents of the workout itself. Jumping straight into exercise is both ineffectual and dangerous. Just as a car needs to be warmed up before it will run smoothly, it takes time for the body to 'get going' and change from normal resting levels to a point at which it is ready to face the rigours of intense exercise.

Because the body tissues are stiffer and less pliable when cold, muscles are more easily pulled and joints can be damaged. In addition, the heart beat is speeded up with a jolt instead of increasing gradually, and can become irregular rather than showing its normal smooth rhythm. These changes affecting the heart can be potentially very serious, especially in an older or less active individual. The function of a warm-up is therefore to prepare the body for action, and in so doing both to reduce the likelihood of injury and to make the subsequent exercise routine more effective.

Warm-up types

A warm-up can be either *passive*, during which the body is heated from the outside, or *active*, where exercise is used to form the heat internally. An example of a passive warm-up is to have a sauna or hot shower, while an active warm-up can be achieved through gentle jogging. Both types can be effective, but are appropriate to different situations.

An active warm-up is the type normally used before exercise, while the passive warm-up is useful when working with an injury, for example before stretching a muscle tightened from a previous strain. From the point of view of injury and rehabilitation, the obvious advantage of the passive warm-up is that it does not require the athlete to move the injured tissues in order to create body heat. Another, often neglected, advantage of the passive warm-up is that it does not significantly use up any of the body's energy supplies. This can be important before competition, when a passive warm-up is used to maintain body heat after an active warm-up has been performed. The major disadvantage of a passive warm-up, however, is that when the body is heated from outside, the heat may not penetrate deep enough to affect the tissues being used in a workout. For example the heat from a standard heat lamp may only penetrate the body by 1 cm. This is fine for superficial muscles, but will not significantly affect the joints. For this to occur either a specialist form of deep heating (diathermy) must be used, or an active warm-up must be chosen.

PREPARATION FOR TRAINING

Effects of a warm-up

A good warm-up will have a number of effects. First, it will make the actions which follow it smoother through *rehearsal*. This is the reasoning behind taking a practice swing before hitting a golf ball, for example, and is useful before any activity which requires *skill*. When we lift a weight or perform any bodytoning action, the movement actually involves dozens of smaller actions all linked together. Muscles must contract at the right time and with the right amount of strength, and joints must move far enough but not too far. These individual components of a movement all come together to form a single action called by scientists a *motor programme*. Each different bodytoning exercise will have a different motor programme, and it is important that a warm-up reminds you of the right sort of motor programme for the exercise you are about to do. Although you are familiar with an exercise when you work out, you will start to forget its technique as soon as you leave the gym. By the time you come back into the gym some days later, you will have performed hundreds of other movements at home and at work, so your gym movements are no longer fresh in your mind. One function of a warm-up is to familiarise you with the motor programme required for an exercise before you use the movement with heavy weights. This is especially important when an exercise uses high speed.

Next, a warm-up will increase your *heart beat* and raise *blood pressure* steadily and safely, rather than causing them to jump dangerously from resting to training levels. This is particularly important in the older or less active individual where the cardiovascular (CV) system of the body may be at risk of injury or disease. Sudden changes in heart rate or blood pressure could put this individual at risk of a heart attack. Throughout the day, at normal resting levels only 15–20 per cent of the total amount of blood in the body goes to the muscles. The rest will be in the body organs. When we exercise however 75 per cent of the blood must be in the working muscles and so we have to divert it from the body organs, and this must be done gradually.

Why warm-up?

In the early 1970s studies were conducted which graphically illustrate the importance of a warm-up to the CV system (Barnard *et al.* 1973). Researchers asked subjects to run vigorously on a treadmill for 10–15 seconds initially *without* a warm-up. In 70% of these subjects, *dangerously abnormal heart beats* were seen using a standard hospital heart rate machine (ECG). These changes were greatly reduced and in most cases not seen at all when the same subjects ran on the treadmill after a warm-up. The researchers also looked at blood pressure, and found that subjects running without a warm-up had a much *higher blood pressure* (168 mmHg) than those who used a warm-up (140 mmHg).

The warmth produced in the body by a warm-up will increase the flow of blood (*local blood flow*) through the tissues and has a number of effects. The contraction and relaxation of muscle is more effective because the chemical reactions involved in this process are speeded up by heating. Similarly the electrical impulses travelling along nerves move faster, and so movements are smoother and less sluggish. Finally, muscles and joints contain fluids which can be stiff. Heating these fluids with a warm-up reduces the stiffness and makes movements easier. All in all warmth makes the body move more effectively.

A *general* warm-up affects the whole body, and should always be followed by a *specific* warm-up that concentrates on the part or parts of the body which will be used in a particular exercise. For example if you are to perform a bench press action (see p. 109), a general warm-up may be on a static cycle or cross training machine. This will warm the body and increase the heart beat, but do little for the arms which will be worked in the bench press action. A specific warm-up for the bench press would involve shoulder, chest and arm movements aiming to stretch the chest (pectoral) muscles and practise a 'pressing' action.

WARM-UP TECHNIQUES

The amount of activity required in a warm-up will depend on a person's fitness level and on the intensity of the exercise or sport to be undertaken. This is because different people raise their body temperature at different rates, depending on body size, amount of body fat and rate of energy metabolism. In addition, different sports will make very different demands on the body's tissues. For this reason the warm-up before a vigorous game of squash, for example, would need to be more extensive than that which might precede a casual round of golf. Equally, a top-level sprinter will require a more thorough warm-up session than a weekend sportsman, because the sprinter is likely to be able to push himself to a higher level of physical activity.

Practically, the warm-up may be practised in three parts: *pulse raising, mobility* and *rehearsal*.

Pulse raising

To be effective, a pulse raising activity should be performed which is intense enough to raise the heart rate (pulse rate) and cause mild sweating. When this happens, the inside (core) temperature of the body has increased by about 1°C. It is best to perform the warm-up wearing a full track suit or other insulating clothing; this keeps in body heat and maintains the benefits of the warm-up until the sport is to be performed. Gentle jogging, light aerobics, or using CV machines in the gym such as static cycles, recumbent cycles, cross trainers, rowers and treadmills are all useful for pulse raising activities.

Mobility

Mobility exercises should be performed sufficient to take the joints through their full range of motion, the exact range being determined by the movements to be used during the workout (see also components of fitness p. 9). The aim is to ensure that the movements used in the workout will not overstretch the tissues. A distinction must be made here between *maintenance stretching* and *developmental stretching*. Maintenance stretches are used prior to a workout to take the tissues to their maximum comfortable range. For developmental stretching, exercises are used which aim to increase this range of motion, and so a thorough warm-up is performed first. In other words maintenance stretches form part of a warm-up, while developmental stretches are practised in a separate stretching session.

Rehearsal

Finally, for complex moves (especially free weight exercises) the specific action of the individual exercise should be rehearsed during the warm-up period. This normally means performing the first set of exercises with a light resistance, or even an unweighted bar or stick. For example when performing a bench press movement, the pin of the machine may be taken out and the exercise performed initially using the first fixed weight alone. For a free weight squatting movement the weight discs may be removed from the bar and the exercise repeated using the bar alone. For a clean and jerk action, a wooden pole may be all that is necessary for the rehearsal portion of the warm-up. For rehearsal, rather than light sweating which indicates that the correct core temperature has been achieved, it is technique which is the deciding factor. Only when the individual can perform the movement correctly has the rehearsal portion of the warm-up achieved its aim.

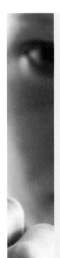

Arousal

In addition to rehearsing an action, there is another mental effect of warm-up, and that is 'arousal'. When we go into a gym after a hard day's work, we may feel lethargic and 'under aroused'. The warm-up may then serve to psyche us up and encourage us to exercise. If we go into an important sports competition however, we may feel 'over aroused' with our heart pumping, palms sweating and that sick feeling in the pit of our stomach. Now, the arousal level is too high, and the appropriate warm-up would actually be to relax and take some time to chill out before we compete. The warm-up then has to prepare us mentally, taking into account our present level of arousal.

WARM-DOWN

Just as it is vital to begin an exercise session slowly, so it is important to end it in the same way. When you exercise hard your heart beat is increased, and the process is actually helped by the contraction of the exercising muscles. This system, known as the 'auxiliary muscle pump', is important to the functioning of the cardiovascular system.

If you stop exercising suddenly, the muscles no longer contract and pump blood along the vessels which travel through them. The demand placed on the heart is greater and the pulse actually increases, even though you have stopped exercising!

A good example of this is provided by the use of electric treadmills in the gym. When inexperienced users run on these they sometimes get carried away, and get faster and faster until they start to become exhausted. Instead of slowing down, they jump off the treadmill in a panic, momentarily increasing the demand on the heart – sometimes with tragic consequences.

Another important feature of the warm-down period is that it can help to reduce muscle ache (see chapter 3) by flushing fresh blood through the muscle used in the workout. Use similar exercises to those chosen for the warm-up. Start the warm-down at the intensity of your workout and gradually slow down until your pulse is back to its normal resting level. In this way you are increasing the blood flow to the muscles which have been worked and taking away the chemicals which cause muscle soreness. Using a warm shower after exercise is a passive way to warm down, as is gentle massage. Both will encourage blood flow through the muscle without working it and so producing even more chemicals.

CLOTHING

Clothing for the gym should be comfortable. Loose-fitting clothes are essential for unrestricted movement, but they should not be so loose that they could get trapped in moving gym machinery. Shorts and T-shirts or a leotard are fine, but fleecy garments should be worn during the warm-up and then removed later as you get hot. Shoes for the gym should support the foot and provide adequate grip while allowing free movement. Training shoes are the obvious choice, but specialist shoes designed for one sport do not necessarily transfer to another. For example, running shoes often restrict the sideways movements of the foot and can be uncomfortable when performing some leg exercises with weights. Whatever shoes you choose, make sure that the laces are kept short so that you do not step on them and trip.

Many people wear different types of joint strapping, the most popular being for the wrist and knee. If you have an injury you should not train except under the direction of your physiotherapist. When recovering from an injury and restrengthening a part of the body, a strapping is not normally used. However, preventive strapping properly applied does have a place if you have a particular weakness which has not responded to treatment. Usually the elastic supports worn in the gym serve two functions. They keep a joint warm, especially if they are made of neoprene; this can be of particular advantage in the case of an arthritic joint. They also offer psychological support by giving the athlete confidence that the joint will not collapse. Provided supports are not used to cover up an injury and work through pain, they are harmless.

Weight training gloves are useful. These are fingerless gloves, usually leather palmed and string backed, or neoprene. They have a padded area over the palm where you grip a weight training bar, and help to prevent the build-up of hard skin which occurs there with regular training. In addition, the padding on the palm of the glove will absorb shock on the hand and wrist, and relax the grip slightly. This is because the fingers' tendons are stretched further when gripping a narrow object and stretched less when gripping a broader object. The size of grip is more important with some elbow conditions such as tennis elbow. The size of grip must feel comfortable and on the whole gripping on a slightly larger area which is spongy is more comfortable than a hard metal bar. Many weight training machines have rotating plastic or rubber handles but free weights do not, making gloves especially important for free weight exercises.

A weight training belt is another piece of equipment which is regaining popularity. These were originally used by weight lifters to protect the lower back when lifting very heavy weights. They are thick leather or reinforced neoprene belts, usually about 10–15 cm wide. Worn around the waist, the stiffness supports the lower spine in two ways: it reminds the user to keep the lower spine flat; and it increases the pressure within the abdomen, which in turn reduces the strain placed on the spinal discs. However, belts will only support the spine if worn tightly, so when you see someone with a bright red belt hanging down loosely over the hips, it is for fashion and not for protection!

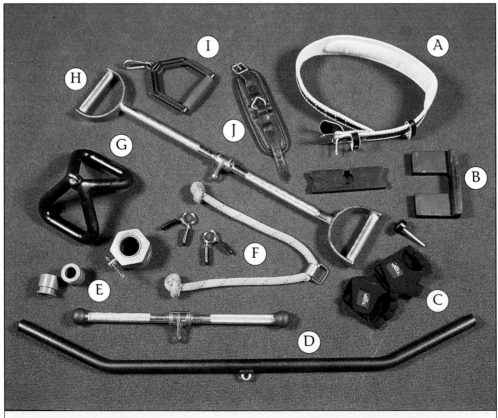

(A) weight training belt, (B) box frame, (C) weight training gloves, (D) lat bar, (E) biceps curl bar, (F) tricep push-down, (G) seated row handle, (H) front lat pull, (I) hexagonal collar, (J) ankle strap

Modern gyms are usually clean, well lit and inviting. Although they look very appealing, however, they contain many potential dangers, and so basic safety standards must always be applied if accidents are to be avoided.

The way you prepare yourself and the care you take with the apparatus are both important. Loose clothing, long hair and dangling jewellery can all catch on the moving parts of weight training machines, taking the user into the apparatus and causing severe injury. Large rings can get caught and slice into your finger. If a sharp ring will not come off, cover it with tape or wear a weight training glove over it.

Exercising in bare feet is not wise. Weights can be dropped and toes can be stubbed. In addition you may step on sharp objects or slip on wooden or rubberised flooring. Thin rubber shoes and flip-flops are little better, and really have no place in the gym even in the height of summer.

Now to the equipment itself. Always check this before use because broken or defective machinery can cause injury. Collars on free weights can work loose and fall off, and

Take off your rings!

Wearing a ring can cause two types of injury, 'laceration' and 'de-gloving'. A laceration occurs when the sharp portion of the ring catches on the user or another person. The momentum of the moving hand causes the sharp ring to cut deeply into the skin tearing as it goes. A de-gloving injury occurs when the ring catches on a piece of moving machinery. The ring cuts into the skin and stays where it is as the hand moves. The result is than some (or all) of the skin is peeled off the finger 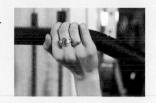 often requiring plastic surgery to repair it. The message is simple, if you are wearing a sharp unprotected ring you should not work out!

stiff machines may be set in motion with a jolt. The weights on solid dumb-bells should always be checked to ensure that they are screwed up tightly before use. When working on free weights it is always better to work with a partner and use a 'buddy' system. Before you lift, your buddy checks your weights and during your lift they check your technique. You do the same for him/her and in this way you are less likely to overlook important safety issues when you are 'psyched up' to lift.

With multi-stack apparatus, make sure the selector key is pushed right into the machine and twisted so that it is locked into place. If pulley cables become snagged, get help; don't try to free them by yourself. Never touch the pulleys and cables when they are in use. Finally, make sure that the machinery is correctly adjusted for your size. It may take a few extra moments to change the settings, but this is time well spent in terms of comfort and safety.

Unfortunately, the spine is at risk when weights are lifted; however, good lifting technique and general care of the back will reduce the likelihood of injury considerably. Dangers come from three sources: poor alignment, repeated bending and fast, uncontrolled movements. If your alignment is optimal (see p. 41) the forces on the joint are minimised and the muscles are worked correctly. With poor alignment joint loading forces are increased, stressing the tissues surround the joint (ligaments and the joint capsule in particular). In addition the muscles may be overstretched (lengthened) or cramped up (shortened) unnecessarily making injury more likely.

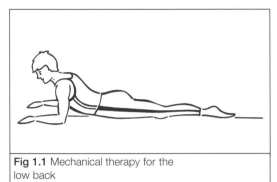

Fig 1.1 Mechanical therapy for the low back

In the case of bending, the discs in the base of the spine are squeezed out of shape and pressed closer to the delicate nerves travelling from the spinal cord to the legs. Repeated bending can cause irritation of these nerves, leading to back pain or sciatica. Try therefore to keep forward bending to a minimum when weight training, and maintain the natural hollow in the base of the spine when standing or sitting to place the spinal discs in their optimal alignment.

During general weight training the spinal discs are compressed and water is squeezed from them. This has the effect of actually shortening the spine after a workout. To help offset this, stretch the spine after training by holding onto the high bar and hanging for between 30 and 60 seconds. It is also useful to include exercises which stretch the spine, such as chin-ups, dips and lateral pull downs, in the latter part of a workout that involves compression exercises (for example, squats and shoulder presses).

Because bending the spine causes problems, arching the spine can help to offset them. This fact enables us to compensate to a certain degree for some of the problems which may occur while training. The following is one of the physiotherapy techniques known as 'mechanical therapy' (Fig. 1.1). Lie on the floor as though you were about to do a push-

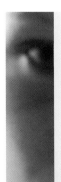

Compression of lumbar discs

Researchers have shown that squat exercises can create compression forces on the lumbar disc of 6–10 times body weight (Cappozzo *et al.* 1985). These forces greatly affect the discs and lead to a dramatic loss in body height. In a 25 minute bout of weight training the average height loss has been shown to be 5.4 mm (Leatt *et al.* 1986) while static loading (standing still with a weight across the shoulders) can lead to a height reduction of 11.2 mm (Tyrrell *et al.* 1985).

up exercise. Keep your legs and hips down on the floor and push up with the arms, arching your spine as you do so. Look forwards, pause momentarily in this position, and then lower yourself down onto the floor again. Repeat this movement ten times. You should find that this starts to relieve any back pain caused through repeated bending. Obviously this exercise is not a 'cure-all', so it is best to avoid repeated bending as much as possible – prevention being better than cure!

Rapid movements, particularly twisting, can also tax the spine. Rapid trunk twisting or bending should be avoided because the weight of the spine and trunk builds up momentum. This momentum will tear at the spinal tissues at the very end of the movement, overstretching them and making them swell. As the swelling forms slowly, you will not actually feel pain until you get up the next morning. Then, your back will be stiff and take time to 'get going'. The best bet in this case is to rest for a few days, and, when you resume training, correct any faulty exercise techniques. If pain still persists, have a word with your physiotherapist.

Table 1.1. Safety check-list for the gym

> Always warm up before training.
> Check machinery before use.
> Set up machinery to suit your body size and weight.
> Tie back long hair and be careful with loose clothing.
> Remove jewellery or place tape over rings which will not come off.
> Wear serviceable footwear – no flip-flops!
> Use correct exercise techniques and keep the weight under control.
> Watch your body alignment – keep a neutral, stable spine.
> Practise good back care – lift correctly.
> Train within your own limitations.
> Never train through an injury – see a physiotherapist.

When lifting free weights from the floor, correct technique is important for protection of the spine. Before you lift, take up a stable position with your feet astride and at least one foot flat. Bend your knees and get down to the level of the weight, keeping your spine hollow as you move. Grip the weight securely, and use the power of your legs, not your back, to lift. As you do this, look up! Bring the weight close into your waist as soon as possible in order to reduce the leverage forces acting on the spine. When you put the weight down, reverse this sequence, always using the strength of your legs and not your back.

THE COMPONENTS OF FITNESS

What is fitness? Is a delicate ballet dancer 'fit' to play in a rugby scrum, or a sumo wrestler 'fit' to run marathons? Common sense tells us that these athletes would not be considered suitable for the alternative sports suggested, and yet most would agree that both top-class ballet dancers and wrestlers are fit.

The answer to this conundrum is that two types of fitness exist: that which is necessary for general health (health-related fitness); and the extreme requirements for excellence at a particular sport or activity (task-related fitness). We can consider the components of fitness as 'S' factors (Fig. 1.2). In the case of general health, three S factors are important: stamina, suppleness and strength.

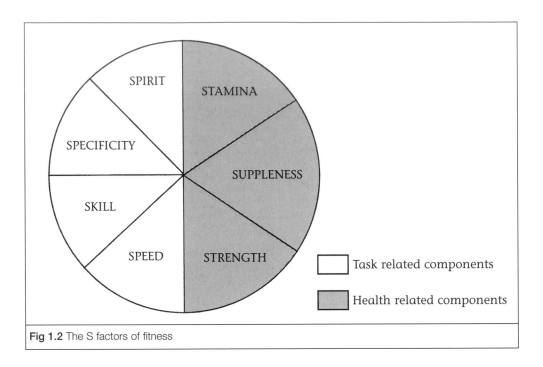

Fig 1.2 The S factors of fitness

HEALTH-RELATED FITNESS

Stamina

Within the term 'stamina' we need to look at both cardiovascular (CV) endurance and local muscle endurance. CV endurance relates to the condition of the heart, lungs and circulation. It describes the ability to keep doing a particular exercise without getting breathless. Exercises that improve CV endurance are rhythmical in nature; examples include fast walking, swimming and cycling, all of which make the heart beat faster and keep it at this rate for some time. This type of exercise strengthens the heart muscle, expands the lungs and conditions the blood vessels, and it is these changes which help to protect an individual from heart problems.

When training to improve CV endurance, three factors are important: how hard an exercise is (intensity); how long it goes on (duration); and how often it is performed (frequency). The intensity of an exercise can be assessed by measuring the heart rate. The maximum heart rate (HRmax) is generally said to be (220 – age) beats/min (see p. 20). In order to gain the benefits of CV endurance training, the heart rate must increase to what is known as the target heart rate (THR); this is a percentage of the age-determined maximum.

There is a trade-off between intensity and duration of exercise. Generally speaking, the harder an exercise is, the less you need to do of it; there are however upper and lower limits of intensity, duration and frequency of training. On average, three periods of CV endurance work are required each week, at an intensity of between 70 and 90 per cent of HRmax. The lower percentage is more suitable for beginners, and exercise of this intensity should be continued for about 30 to 40 minutes. Higher intensities will suit the more experienced athletes, and need only be carried out for 20 to 30 minutes. If a person simply runs 'flat out' for 2 minutes the intensity of the exercise is sufficient, but the exercise will not have been kept up for long enough to allow the necessary changes to occur in the body. Similarly, a casual stroll around the park may be of a sufficient duration, but the exercise intensity is too low.

It is also important to realise that the duration of the CV endurance training refers only to the aggregate of the times at which the heart beat is high. It does not refer to the duration of the workout itself. You may spend 40 minutes in the gym, but possibly half of this time is spent resting or waiting for apparatus to become free. The heart rate will reduce in these periods and they will not count towards improving your CV endurance.

Local muscle endurance is improved by working muscles against low resistances over a longer period. The aim is to improve the ability of the muscle to work largely without oxygen. To do this the amount of lactic acid which is formed in the muscle (see p. 16) is a deciding factor. The more tolerance an individual can build up to the accumulation of lactic acid, the greater the local muscle endurance. In general, the intensity of muscle endurance training is low, but the duration high. The amount of weight that can be lifted in a single repetition is measured (the 'one repetition maximum' or 1RM) and exercises are performed as a percentage of this amount. For endurance weights at 10–20 per cent 1RM may be used, but for higher numbers of repetitions 15–25 repetitions is normally the minimum to be used in weight training. For circuit weight training, times of 30–90 seconds may be used. The relationship between strength, endurance and repetition number is covered on p. 88 – and the principles behind circuit weight training (CWT) on p. 162.

Suppleness

This refers to the amount of movement at a joint, and is an important factor in determining its health. Suppleness exercises are slow and controlled. They move a joint through its full range of motion so you feel the 'stretch'.

Three types of stretching are generally used: static, ballistic and neuromuscular. Static stretching is the type used in yoga for example. The fully stretched position is held, and any tightness gradually subsides.

Ballistic stretching is often used in sport and involves adding small 'bounces' when at the fully stretched position in an attempt to extend the range of movement still further. This type of stretching can be dangerous if the small bounces become large and uncontrolled. This is a specialist type of stretching not suitable for the beginner. It should only be performed under the supervision of a physiotherapist or experienced personal trainer. It is vital that the bounces are small controlled oscillations rather than rapid uncontrolled swinging at the end of range.

The third type of stretching, termed neuromuscular, uses the muscle reflexes. When a muscle is contracted and held (isometric contraction) the muscle tone relaxes below resting level as the contraction is released. During this period a stretch may effectively be put on to perform Contract Relax (CR) stretching. Using another muscle reflex, when a

PREPARATION FOR TRAINING

Holding static stretches

Research has shown that the optimal holding time for a static stretch is longer than previously thought (Bandy and Irion 1994). Comparing holding times of 15, 30 and 60 seconds, the 30s hold gave a better improvement in stretching but the 60s hold did not improve this any further. It seems that a prolonged 30s stretch is more effective, but a stretch longer than this is no better. Other researchers have looked at the number of repetitions (Taylor *et al.* 1990) and found that 4–5 reps is optimal. More reps does not give any additional benefit. Performing 5 reps of a static stretch and holding each for 30 seconds will give the best results.

muscle contracts its neighbour on the other side of the joint (the antagonist) relaxes and the stretch can again be put on to better effect. Using these two types of stretching on the hamstring muscles, for example, tighten them first by slightly bending the knee against resistance and then allow them to relax (CR) before stretching. After this has been performed a number of times, tighten the quadriceps muscles (antagonists to the hamstrings) to straighten the knee and you will find the stretch goes further. For further information on stretching see my book *The Complete Guide to Stretching*, A&C Black, 1999.

When any part of the body is stretched, two types of tissue are affected: contractile tissue (muscle); and non-contractile tissue (ligaments, tendons, joint capsules, etc.). Normally it will be the muscles that limit the movement, and so the muscle stretching techniques described above are used. After injury, however, the non-contractile structures may tighten. When stretching these, basic mechanical principles apply – the tissue will become more pliable when heated. This may be partially achieved through an active or passive warm-up. When stretching a tight ligament or joint capsule after an injury, a physiotherapist may use a form of heating called short-wave diathermy to convey heat deep into the joint and so make stretching the previously injured tissues much easier. The principles of tissue warming are the same; only the method has changed.

TASK-RELATED FITNESS

In addition to general fitness, sports performance requires 'task-related' fitness components, particularly speed, skill, specificity and spirit. These are not related to general health in the same way as stamina, suppleness and strength. They are however important in the prevention of sports injuries and the safe return to sport after injury.

Speed

Speed and power are trained through fast, explosive actions. When a movement is performed quickly, for example, a rapid running action, we are developing speed. If a fast action is performed against a resistance, for example, a piece of weight training apparatus, we are training for power. Fast actions build up a lot of momentum, and are therefore difficult to stop. This is an important safety consideration in the case of power training, and power exercises must always be controlled and executed with good technique. Athletes training for power frequently 'pre-stretch' a muscle (i.e. stretch it immediately before contracting it); in this way they utilise the elastic properties of the muscle to overcome a greater resistance. This is the basis of plyometric training (see p. 190).

Skill

A skilled action will be made up of a number of individual movement components strung together to form a sequence called a 'motor programme'. Forming this motor programme takes time and the individual has to progress through three distinct phases before the skill is mastered. The first stage is to understand what the movement entails and for this to happen the individual must 'feel' the movement. As it goes wrong, this must be corrected by close supervision and coaching before enough skill has been built up for unsupervised practice to be safe. This is the stage of swimming where a person is still thrashing in the pool with 'doggy paddle'. In terms of weight training it is the stage when a person has just been shown how to do a bench press action, for example, and has tried it once or twice but is unable to remember all the teaching points of the exercise. Once an exercise has been practised we move into the second stage of skill learning called the 'motor phase'. Now the individual can perform the action and knows what to do. However, they still need to concentrate closely on the skill and it does not yet flow freely. They still need some coaching but are now able to identify their own mistakes so are safe to work alone. With lots more practice the skill becomes second nature and we have moved into the third stage of skill learning called the 'associative phase'. Now the action virtually runs by itself. This is the stage we are in when we drive. We no longer have to think about changing gear as it has become second nature. Skills which have developed to this stage can be performed rapidly with little thought.

Specificity

There are really two aspects to this component. In terms of exercise physiology, specificity refers to the SAID principle, standing for Specific Adaptation to Imposed Demand. This really means that the changes which take place in the body (the adaptation) are very closely related, or specific, to the exercise we use (the imposed demand). For example, an isometric exercise for the arm performed with the arm at 90° will develop the greatest amount of strength with the arm joint at this right-angled position. If we were to measure the arm strength with the elbow held at positions of more or less than a right-angle, we would find the strength gain to be inferior. This holds true for fitness components other than strength. Although running marathons and doing sprint training will both make you fitter, the changes that take place within the body will be completely different in each case.

PREPARATION FOR TRAINING

The other meaning of the term 'specificity' encompasses those fitness components which are unique to a sport but may not necessarily be good for the sportsman's health. For example, a high body weight is important in sumo wrestling; a high degree of flexibility can be required in certain types of ballet and in gymnastics. Athletes wishing to excel at these particular sports will require these specific fitness components, but clearly neither excessive body weight nor excessive flexibility are good for a person's health.

If you are using weight training to enhance your performance at a particular sport, it is important that you take some time to work out the specific aspects of fitness that your sport demands. Developing the wrong ones will not just waste your time, but may also lower your performance standard!

Spirit

The term spirit here is used to represent the psychological aspects of exercise. Within this term are included items such as arousal level (p. 4), which is important during warm-up, and goal setting (p. 104), an important aspect of exercise planning and motivation. Spirit is also important after injury, where exercise can be used not just to improve the strength and flexibility of a limb, but also to rebuild a person's confidence in using it. This is especially true after serious injuries such as fractures, for example.

BODYTONING

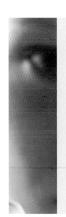

In order to exercise we need energy or fuel in much the same way as a car engine does. We get our fuel from the food that we eat. Food is broken down by the digestive system and the goodness or *nutrients* that are released are taken in the bloodstream to the working muscles. Here, the nutrients react with chemical substances called *enzymes* to release the energy that enables us to exercise. Some foodstuffs provide more energy than others. For example, sugars and fats are high energy providers, while fibre is a very low energy source.

When broken down, the energy from the food is stored by special chemicals called *phosphates*. These high-energy phosphate fuels can be thought of as the 'petrol' in the body's 'engine'.

ENERGY SOURCES

Phosphates are our energy 'currency', and we can 'spend' them in three ways when exercising. This gives us a choice of immediate, short term or long term energy supplies.

ATP

One of the most important phosphate substances is *adenosine triphosphose* or ATP. This acts as a link between the processes supplying energy and those (such as muscle contraction) which demand it. ATP is composed of a nitrogen substance called *adenine* linked to a sugar called *ribose* and three phosphate molecules. When one phosphate molecule is removed from ATP, *adenosine diphosphate* (ADP) is produced and energy is released.

Immediate energy sources

A muscle can only store enough energy in the form of phosphate for about 5 seconds of maximal work. The phosphate in this case comes as a special substance called *phospho-creatine* (PC). This energy source, although used up quickly, is readily available, because it does not take time to 'switch on'. It enables us to react quickly and work maximally straightaway, rather than waiting for our energy to build up.

For example, PC is used in the first few seconds of a sprint and during a low number of maximal repetitions in weight training. It is the energy source for power and speed rather than prolonged strength or endurance activities.

Short-term energy sources (the lactic acid system)

If exercise continues the PC stores will quickly deplete, forcing a muscle to use sugars (glycogen) for energy. This new process is termed *glycolysis*, and enables the muscle to continue to perform intense work – but at a price. The price is *lactic acid,* formed as a waste product, which interferes with the working of the muscle. This causes the muscle to ache, and continuing the exercise eventually becomes too painful. The build-up of lactic acid is one of the sources of the 'burn' that is familiar to many sportsmen.

The build-up of lactic acid limits the usefulness of this short-term energy supply to about two minutes. Normally, at rest the concentration of lactic acid in the body is about 2 units for every kilogram of muscle tissue. After heavy exercise, this concentration may increase to as much as 25 units as fatigue sets in.

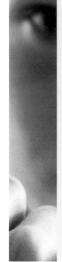

Lactate accumulation curve

As the intensity of short-term exercise increases, the amount of lactic acid (lactate) in the blood increases proportionally. A graph of lactate plotted against exercise intensity (*the lactate accumulation curve*) shows a smooth line, with two distinct changes in gradient or 'breaks'. The first break in the curve is called the *lactate threshold* and is seen at exercise intensities of 50–60% of maximum. The second break, called the *Onset of Blood Lactate Accumulation* (OBLA) appears at intensities of 70–80% maximum. The breaks reflect the changes in use of different sizes and types of muscle fibres (see p. 27). With training the curve moves to the right, meaning that the amount of lactate formed with a particular exercise is less as you get fitter (Fig. 2.1). Less lactate means less aching and the ability to exercise for longer – your muscle endurance has therefore improved.

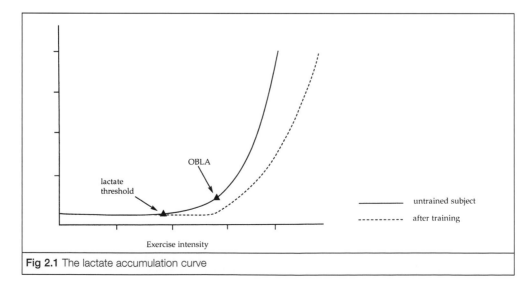

Fig 2.1 The lactate accumulation curve

Both glycolysis and the PC system supply energy without using oxygen and are therefore described as *anaerobic*. For longer term energy used in endurance events we need to produce the energy more effectively. To do this we must combine the food nutrients with oxygen from the air. When this happens energy is said to be supplied *aerobically*.

Long-term energy sources (the oxygen system)

Several fuels can be broken down in the presence of oxygen to form energy aerobically. These fuels include sugars, fats and even protein in some cases. As these substances are broken down, their energy is transferred to the body's high-energy phosphates, especially ATP. This process is slower than both glycolysis and the PC system, and it may be 2–3 minutes before the energy needs of the body cells are met.

During this time the body, which is supplying its tissues with enough oxygen for resting requirements, must take measures to meet its increased needs during exercise. Heart and breathing rates increase, breathing becomes deeper, and the blood flow to the working muscles improves. When all these changes have stabilised, you are said to have reached a *steady state*.

With training, these changes occur more rapidly because the systems involved become stronger. This is one of the health benefits of regular exercise. People in poor physical condition tend to take longer to reach steady state because their heart, lungs and muscles are not as efficient as those of trained athletes. A comparison between the three energy systems is shown in Figure 2.2.

In practice, the three systems work hand in hand. For example, when you start to exercise, the PC system and glycolysis will supply the energy initially. The aerobic processes will take slightly longer to come on line. In addition, the aerobic system will not stop immediately on cessation of exercise, but will continue to work for a short while to recharge the other two energy sources. During this period lactic acid and other waste products are removed from the tissues so that they are ready for the next exercise period.

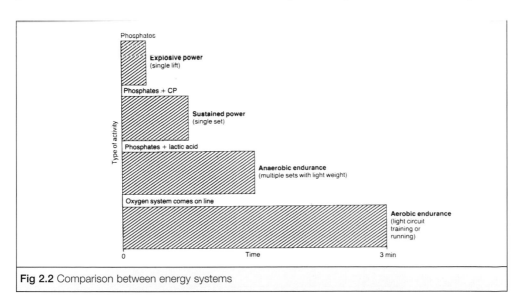

Fig 2.2 Comparison between energy systems

Oxygen from the air has to be taken into the body and then to the working muscle cells. The oxygen is breathed in by the lungs and carried by the bloodstream to the body cells. In order to understand the changes that occur during exercise it is necessary to look briefly at the various stages of this pathway.

The pulmonary system

We require more oxygen during exercise than we do when we are sedentary; in a vigorous workout we can increase our need for oxygen by as much as 25 times. In order to get more oxygen we must take in a larger quantity of air. Normally, when we sit quietly relaxing, only a small portion of the lungs is working. Breathing movements are restricted to the upper parts of the lungs, and some of the lung areas are completely shut off.

Air is taken in through the nose and mouth and into the windpipe. This branches into the left and right lung, and then each branch divides again and again into millions of very fine air tubes. At the end of each tube a tiny balloon-like airsack (*the alveolus*) fills with air as we breathe in and empties as we breathe out. The airsacks provide a huge surface area; in fact, if they were all flattened out they would cover a whole badminton court! The tubes can be opened or closed by surrounding muscles, and in this way the body can control which areas of the lungs are working at any one time.

Asthma

During an asthma attack the muscles surrounding the air tubes go into spasm, trapping air in the airsacks. If this happens to an athlete who is not used to it, he or she must be told to relax and breathe slowly. If the athlete panics and starts to gasp for air, trying to force the lungs to work, the situation will only get worse.

The lungs are enclosed in the rib cage, which is a little like a barrel. The floor of the barrel is a sheet of muscle called the *diaphragm*. As we breathe in, two things happen to the chest cavity. First, the diaphragm lowers, pulling the floor of the cavity downwards. Second, the ribs, which are attached to the breastbone at the front and to the spine at the back, open up expanding the walls of the chest cavity. The combination of rib and diaphragm movement increases the size of the chest cavity and pulls air into the lungs. As we breathe out, the process is reversed, and the elasticity of the chest structures and lung airsacks forces air out again (see Fig. 2.3).

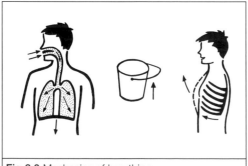

Fig 2.3 Mechanics of breathing

In heavy smokers the airsacks are less elastic, expansion of the lungs is restricted and the person therefore finds it difficult to take in sufficient air.

During exercise, additional muscles are used to expand the rib cage. These accessory muscles of respiration include those of the chest, neck and rib cage and can be seen working when a person runs flat out.

Movement of the ribs

Two types of rib movement occur when we breath in, called *pump handle* and *bucket handle* actions. Pump handle movement is seen when the breastbone (sternum) lifts up and out. This type of movement is often restricted with a round shouldered posture where the chest is flattened in a front to back direction. Bucket handle movement occurs as the ribs expand by flaring sideways. This increases the diameter of the rib cage and is often restricted when only small shallow breaths are taken.

The oxygen transport system

Once air has been taken into the airsacks, oxygen moves across the moist airsack walls and into small blood vessels. From here it is taken in the blood to join the nutrients from the food in the working muscle. Carbon dioxide travels the reverse route, from the working muscle in the bloodstream and across the airsack wall. It is then expelled from the lungs and breathed out.

Oxygen is carried in the blood by a substance called *haemoglobin* contained within the red blood cells. Oxygen-rich blood is red and is carried by the main arteries into smaller blood vessels and capillaries, eventually passing into the body cells themselves. Blood containing carbon dioxide has a blue tinge and is carried in the veins back to the lungs to be breathed back into the atmosphere.

Haemoglobin is rich in iron. People with anaemia have too little haemoglobin and therefore too little iron, and this deficiency impedes their sporting performance. Athletes who train at high altitudes (where the air is 'thinner') have more haemoglobin and red blood cells than others because their body adapts to the lower concentration of available oxygen. This is why athletes competing in countries that are situated at a great distance above sea-level have to spend a period of time before their event training at high altitude. This is known as *acclimatisation*.

With training in general, the body improves its ability to transport and use oxygen for the supply of energy. Fit people therefore have more haemoglobin and a greater number of small blood capillaries in their muscles than unfit people. In addition, their lungs and heart are more powerful so they can get a greater amount of oxygen to their muscles and get it there more quickly.

As we breathe, not all the oxygen is extracted from the air. Room air normally contains about 21 per cent oxygen and a little carbon dioxide. Air that is breathed out

ENERGY SYSTEMS

still contains about 14 per cent oxygen and 6 per cent carbon dioxide. This is why breathing in a confined space, and so not getting enough oxygen, makes you sleepy. For example, a lot of people having a meeting in a small room with poor ventilation will often feel they cannot concentrate and may have a 'thick head' at the end of the day. Because more oxygen is used during exercise, good ventilation is even more important – windows should be open in the gym!

THE CARDIOVASCULAR SYSTEM

The heart is really two pumps joined into one. The left side of the heart transports oxygenated blood from the lungs to the working tissues. The right side of the heart takes the blood containing waste carbon dioxide (deoxygenated blood) from the working tissues back to the lungs.

Heart rate and pulse

The amount of blood pumped by the heart will be determined both by the rate of beating (heart rate or pulse) and by the 'power' of each beat, or the amount of blood that is forced out with each heart-muscle contraction. The blood normally takes approximately one minute to circulate around the body, but during exercise (because the strength of each heart beat and the pulse rate are both increased) this time is dramatically reduced, so the same blood will travel around the body up to six times in a minute.

During exercise, then, the heart must beat faster to meet the oxygen requirements of the working body. There is however a limit to how fast it can beat, and the maximum speed reduces with age. You can work out your maximum rate roughly by using the following equation: maximum heart rate = 220 beats/minute – (minus) your age. A 24-year-old would therefore have a theoretical maximum heart rate of 196 beats per minute.

In addition to beating faster during exercise, the heart will also push out more blood each time it beats. The heart is a muscle, and will react to training by getting stronger in the same way as other muscles. A fit individual will have a big, strong heart that is able to pump large volumes of blood. At rest, the heart will not need to pump as quickly, and so the resting heart beat or pulse will be lower. Normally the pulse is about 70 beats per minute; in fit people it can reduce to 60; and in the case of marathon runners it can even go as low as 40 beats per minute because with each beat so much more blood is pushed out by the heart.

Blood pressure

Another measure of the efficiency of the cardiovascular system is the blood pressure (BP). This is represented by two figures: the first, the *systolic* BP, represents the power of the heart in pushing out blood and will increase during exercise; the second, the *diastolic* BP, reflects the elasticity of the main blood vessels leading from the heart. As the heart pumps blood into these vessels they stretch; as the heart relaxes the vessels spring back. The pressure caused by this elastic recoil is the diastolic BP. This figure will be higher in less fit individuals, as their blood vessels will be more rigid and have less 'give'.

Average blood pressure is 120/80 mmHg. Blood pressures recorded during isometric work, in which the muscles tense and stay contracted, are higher than those recorded during dynamic (moving) work, in which the muscles contract and relax rhythmically. In the case of isometric work, as the resistance to blood flow is increased the muscle contracts and holds, causing a corresponding elevation in blood pressure. During dynamic work, the rhythmic pumping action actually helps the passage of blood through the muscles, and so lower blood pressures are recorded.

ENERGY FROM THE DIET

We have seen that oxygen is combined with digested foodstuffs to supply energy for the working muscles. Now, we need to look at these foodstuffs to discover which foods are better at supplying energy and why.

Carbohydrates

These are commonly called starches or sugars, and are composed of carbon, hydrogen and oxygen in varying proportions. They provide the bulk (substance), and sweetness of most foods such as cereals, fruit, pasta, biscuits and cakes.

Basic carbohydrate units

The basic carbohydrate unit is the *monosaccharide*, of which the simple sugars glucose, fructose and galactose are examples. Two monosaccharides joined together make a *disaccharide*, such as sucrose (or table sugar) which is a combination of glucose and fructose. Other disaccharides include lactose (glucose plus galactose), which is found in milk, and maltose (two glucose molecules joined together), which is produced when starch is broken down. When three or more monosaccharide units are joined together they form a *polysaccharide*. Polysaccharides are used to store glucose for future use as energy. Starch is the polysaccharide found in plants, while glycogen is the polysaccharide used for storage in animals.

A healthy diet is one in which the proportion of refined carbohydrate (monosaccharides and disaccharides) found in sweet foods such as biscuits, chocolate and snacks is reduced, and the proportion of starchy foods containing complex carbohydrates (polysaccharides) such as pasta, potatoes and grains is increased. In addition to having a high polysaccharide content, foods rich in complex carbohydrates also contain the vitamins and minerals necessary for the body to use the carbohydrate. Foods containing large amounts of refined carbohydrate are highly processed and often contain fewer vitamins and minerals; they are therefore less nutritious (see Table 2.1).

Table 2.1 Carbohydrate-rich foods	
Complex carbohydrates (starchy foods – eat more)	**Simple sugars** (refined foods – eat less)
Wholemeal bread Brown rice and pasta Pulses, beans, peas Potatoes, root vegetables Cereals made from wholegrains Fresh fruit	Sugars, jams, toffee Sugary drinks (squashes, lemonade) Malted drinks Jellies, ice cream, sweet custard

When carbohydrates are digested, the energy they release is stored as the substance *glucose*, carried in the blood (also termed blood sugar) and *glycogen* within the muscle. Foods may be classified not just by the type of carbohydrate they contain, but the effect that this carbohydrate has on the body's energy supply. The *Glycaemic Index* (GI) is a method of classifying foods depending on how high they raise the concentration of glucose in the blood and how long they keep it high. The glucose supplied by normal white bread is used as the starting point or *reference value* and given the score of 100. Other foods are then scored in comparison with this value. Foods which give an instant 'high', that is they are digested quickly, and rapidly raise blood sugar levels have a high GI. Those which take longer to digest and increase blood glucose more slowly have a lower GI score. For example, a sugary doughnut has a GI of 108 while a rye bread has a GI of 48.

The GI is determined by a number of factors involved with digestion and absorption of the foodstuff. Foods that are high in fibre tend to slow the blood glucose rise while those which are higher in fat or protein take longer to digest and absorb. Fatty, high protein or fibrous foods therefore tend to have a lower GI, while fat free foods have a higher GI. Foods which have been cooked longer, and nuts, seeds or grains which have been milled or ground, produce a faster rise in blood glucose and therefore have a higher GI (see Table 2.2)

Immediately before training or immediately afterwards we need energy and we need it fast. This is the time to pick the high GI foods. Have some of these in a kit bag or fridge for when you get home so that they are readily available. A bowl of cereal with a banana chopped on top is a good choice. About four hours before a workout (lunchtime if it is an early evening workout) we need slow release energy so that it is still available when we actually exercise. At this time we should choose moderate or low GI foods such as pasta, pulses and soft fruit.

Energy from protein and fat

Protein is the building block of muscle, and fat is a long-term energy store (see page 17). However, both may be used as forms of energy by 'burning' them with oxygen, a process called protein and fat *oxidation*. Fat is broken down by an enzyme (lipase) into smaller units called *triglycerides*. These then react with the oxygen to form energy in much the same way as carbohydrates do. Proteins can be broken down and used as energy when other sources (fats and carbohydrates) are not available. The protein is broken into its component parts (amino acid molecules) and then used.

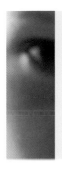

Protein use in exercise

In short-term exercise little protein is used providing other energy sources are on hand. In long-term extreme exercise such as marathon running and triathlon as much as 18% of the energy requirement may come from protein (Brook 1987), a fact that must be given consideration when planning a training diet.

Fluids and electrolytes

Water is probably the most important single component of the diet. Most of the body's tissues are composed mainly of water, which transports vital substances around the body. Water also plays an important role in temperature regulation. Heat formed by the working tissues during exercise is transported to the body surface and lost to the outside. Sweat is excreted onto the skin and evaporates, cooling the body in the process. During intense exercise, especially on a windy day, fluid loss can be excessive. Athletes training hard in such conditions should drink small amounts of water throughout the training period: large amounts taken in one 'gulp' lead to a bloated feeling and may cause a stitch.

During the fluid-loss process, substances called *electrolytes* (mainly salt and potassium) are lost. It is thought that this may contribute to muscle cramps, and so many athletes use electrolyte drinks during training. However, it is doubtful whether these are of marked benefit, and those containing a lot of sugar or salt should be avoided as they may actually inhibit fluid absorption. Athletes training regularly in a hot environment may show significant electrolyte loss in sweat however, and so should ensure that they eat some salty foods and foods rich in potassium (for example, bananas) as a preventive measure.

Some people find drinking dilute fruit juices more palatable than plain tap water. Fruit juice diluted in this way will also provide energy in the form of carbohydrate (fructose). This will be of little value in short-term events, but has been shown to help in endurance events longer than one hour (Below *et al.* 1995).

Table 2.2 The glycaemic index of various foods (glucose – 100)								
High (60 – 100)	**GI**	**Moderate (40 – 60)**	**GI**	**Low (< 40)**	**GI**
Cereals		**Cereals**		**Pulses**	
White bread	69	Wholemeal pasta	42	Butter beans	36
Wholemeal bread	72	White pasta	50	Baked beans	40
Brown rice	80	Oats	49	Haricot beans	31
White rice	82	Barley	22	Chick peas	36
				Lentils	29
				Kidney beans	29
				Soya beans	15
Breakfast cereals		**Breakfast cereals**			
Cornflakes	80	Porridge	54		
Muesli	66	All Bran	51		
Shredded Wheat	67				
Weetabix	75				
Fruit		**Fruit**		**Fruit**	
Raisins	64	Grapes	44	Apples	39
Bananas	62	Oranges	40	Cherries	23
				Plums	25
				Apricots	30
				Grapefruit	26
				Peaches	29
Vegetables		**Vegetables**		**Dairy products**	
Sweetcorn	59	Sweet potatoes	48	Milk	32
Parsnips	97	Crisps	51	Yoghurt	36
Baked potato	98	Yams	51	Ice cream	36
Carrots	92				
Other		**Other**		**Other**	
Biscuits	59	Oatmeal biscuits	54	Fructose	20
Chocolate bar	68	Sponge cake	46		
Honey	87				
Sucrose	59				
Glucose	100				
Orange cordial	66				
From Bean (1997).					

HOW MUSCLES WORK ❮

The human body has in excess of 430 muscles, and if we want to increase bodytone by strengthening and shaping these muscles with weight training, we need to know how they work. The underpinning knowledge of muscle structure and function will enable us to create more effective exercise programmes that are firmly based on science rather than simply hearsay.

STRUCTURE OF A MUSCLE

If we were to take a small piece of muscle out of the body and magnify it many times, we would see that it is made up of many thin fibres. The fibres are grouped together and bound by a membrane, a little like a stack of pencils wrapped in plastic film. The group (called a *fasciculus*), may contain up to 150 individual fibres each about the same diameter as a human hair.

Musculo-tendinous unit

The muscle membranes run the full length of the muscle itself and are continuous with the tendon on the end of the muscle. This means that tension or strength developed by the muscle fibres as they contract is transmitted directly from the centre (belly) of the muscle to the tendon to produce movement. This immediate transmission of force makes the system very efficient. The combination of muscle, muscle membrane, and tendon is referred to as the *musculo-tendinous unit*.

Because stronger muscle pulls harder, the muscle membranes will actually become stronger with training, making them less likely to be injured by strenuous sport, for example. Light aerobics will increase the rate of chemical activity (*metabolism*) in the muscle membranes, while intense weight training will cause the membrane tissue to grow, becoming tougher and thicker. The muscle membranes are also important in supplying elastic strength (p. 30). Because they are very pliable, they will recoil like an elastic band when stretched. This creates force which is in addition to that created by actual muscle contraction.

The nerve controlling the muscle (called a *motor nerve*) touches the muscle fibres at a point called the nerve-muscle or *neuromuscular junction*. Each fibre has only one neuromuscular junction, but a motor nerve may be in contact with several fibres. The combination of muscles fibres and motor nerve is called the *motor unit*.

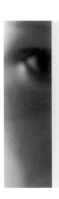

The muscle membrane which surrounds the individual muscle cells (called the *sarcolemma*) has a special property and that is to conduct tiny electrical impulses, a little like a cable joining a light switch to a bulb. The membrane travels right into the inside of the muscle, taking with it the electrical impulses from the nerves on the muscle surface. The connection between the outside and inside of the muscle is through a system of fine channels called 'T-tubules'. The T-tubules have a small sac at their opening which contains calcium, a substance vital to the process of muscle contraction.

Looking at each muscle fibre through a microscope we can see many thousands of exceptionally fine sub-fibres or *myofibrils*, each about 1/100th the width of a human hair. These show alternating light and dark bands corresponding to the different muscle proteins responsible for muscle movement or *contraction.*

Myofibrils

The light area of the small myofibril is composed of a thin filament called *actin* while the dark area consists of a thicker filament called *myosin*. The two sets of filaments fit together like the fingers on two opposing hands. One set of actin-myosin fibres is together called a *sarcomere*. The sarcomere is so small that between 4000 and 5000 would fit together per centimetre. The thick myosin filament has projections or crossbridges coming from it much like the oars of a boat. The thin actin filament has a long filament *(tropomyosin)* wound around it and a smaller globe-shaped molecule *(troponin)* positioned close to it. At rest the tropomyosin prevents (inhibits) actin and myosin from binding.

MUSCLE CONTRACTION

Contraction of the muscle occurs when the muscle filaments move towards each other and a whole sequence of events is required for this to take place. When we want a muscle to contract, a nervous impulse is sent from the brain. This signal travels down the spinal cord and along a nerve to the muscle where it causes a change in the muscle membrane. At the point where the nerve touches the muscle a chemical *(acetylcholine)* is released which causes an electrical impulse to spread across the muscle surface. This in turn causes calcium release from the sacs at the end of the muscle tubules. The calcium is spread into the muscle allowing contraction to occur.

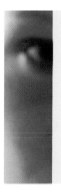

Calcium release

The release of calcium causes the spiral tropomyosin unit to move deeper into the groove of the actin filament removing the inhibition that has been preventing contraction. Once the inhibition has been removed, contraction will occur spontaneously and the muscle filaments pull closer together, causing them to slide over each other and shorten the muscle.

The whole muscle contraction process uses energy and rest is needed to recharge the structures involved. Calcium has to be moved out of the muscle tubule and back into its sac. The filaments must then return to their original relaxed positions.

STRENGTH AND MUSCLE FIBRE TYPE

Not all muscle fibres are of the same type. Some are designed to contract over and over again without fatiguing. These are known as, *slow-twitch* (type I) fibres and have a reddish appearance; they are found in higher concentration in the muscles that control posture, for example, the soleus muscle of the calf. Others, which appear white, are called *fast-twitch* fibres (type II). These give short bursts of power, such as that required in sprinting, but they will fatigue more quickly than the slow-twitch type. An example of a muscle with a large number of fast-twitch fibres is the gastrocnemius in the calf.

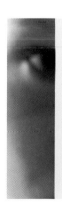

Slow and fast twitch muscles

The names 'slow-' and 'fast-' twitch refer to the firing frequency of the muscle fibre – that is, how many small contractions (twitches) they will produce each second. Slow-twitch fibres produce 10–30 twitches per second while fast-twitch ones produce 30–70. Although the slow and fast fibres are termed type I and type II respectively, there are a number of sub-divisions of fibre types including type IIa and IIb which show intermediate characteristics.

As well as the type of muscle fibres found, the size of the fibre is also important. Small diameter fibres may be brought on line *(recruited)* easily. They are the slow-twitch fibres and are used regularly at effort levels of up to 30 per cent of the maximum. Larger diameter fibres are fast-twitch, and are harder to recruit. They will only be used

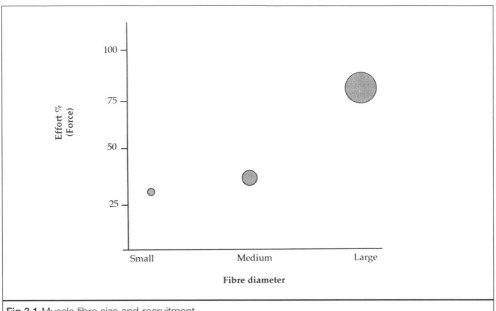

Fig 3.1 Muscle fibre size and recruitment

with efforts greater than 40 per cent of maximum so an individual will have to work quite hard to use these fibres. The very largest diameter fibres however will stay inactive until efforts of as much as 80 per cent maximum are used. These fibres are only used in periods of extreme need, meaning that some people never actually use them with light training programmes. These fibres will be used in maximum poundages in weight training, and are the type used by bodybuilders. Because these fibres are larger in diameter, larger poundages used to successfully recruit them will cause muscles to thicken and build up *(hypertrophy)*. Those wanting to build larger muscles or 'bulk up' should therefore exercise at higher intensities while those wishing to 'tone' should avoid very heavy weights and instead use moderate poundages for higher numbers of repetitions (Fig. 3.1).

ARRANGEMENT OF MUSCLE FIBRES

When a muscle fibre contracts, it shortens and pulls in order to create force. The two actions of creating force and shortening are seen in all muscle fibres, but the arrangement of the fibres within a muscle will dictate whether the muscle is better at shortening to create a large range of motion or pulling to create large forces. A muscle fibre can only shorten by half of its length. If a muscle fibre is longer to begin with it will produce a greater range of motion. An example of a muscle with long fibres is the hamstring at the back of the thigh. The fibres are all in line with each other and they stretch the full length of the muscle, attaching to tendons at each end. This arrangement of fibres is called *parallel* (Fig. 3.2a). If we want greater strength in a muscle, we need more fibres contracting at the same time. If we simply made the muscle bigger it would be too bulky and unwieldy. To achieve increased strength without bulk, the strength-designed muscle connects its fibres to a central tendon in an arrangement called *pennate* (Fig. 3.2b). An example of a pennate muscle is the quadriceps on the front of the thigh. Because each of the muscle fibres is shorter the amount of movement produced is not as great as with the

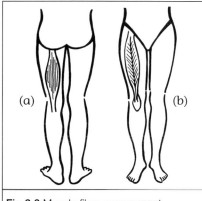

Fig 3.2 Muscle fibre arrangement

parallel muscle, but the far greater number of fibres makes the muscle much stronger.

When weight training, it is important to be aware of the underlying muscle structure so that you can devise more effective programmes. For example, the hamstrings respond well to fast and explosive plyometric training because they are very long and elastic (see p. 189). If heavy weights and slow movements are used to train them they will still get stronger, but they are more likely to be injured when subjected to rapid sprinting and lunging movements.

MUSCLE LENGTH AT REST, AND CONTRACTION SPEED

Two other factors are important with reference to strength and muscle fibres: the resting length of the muscle; and the speed of its movement.

A muscle is strongest when it is contracted from a resting (stretched) state (see Fig. 3.3). If the muscle is shortened, less tension can be exerted because an overlap of the muscle filaments interferes with the contraction. If the muscle is overstretched, the filaments are pulled apart and no tension through contraction can be exerted. For maximum strength then, we should aim to contract a muscle from a comfortably stretched state, and this interaction is known as the *length–tension relationship*. It can be used when training. For example, when trying to lift a heavy weight on a bench press, the bar should be taken down onto the chest in order to place a comfortable stretch on the pectoral muscles. This is more effective than starting from a mid-range position with the bar held off the chest.

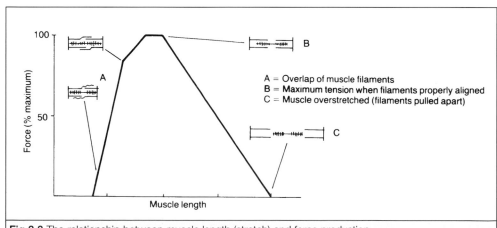

A = Overlap of muscle filaments
B = Maximum tension when filaments properly aligned
C = Muscle overstretched (filaments pulled apart)

Fig 3.3 The relationship between muscle length (stretch) and force production

When a muscle is stretched, however, although less tension can be created by contraction of the muscle, more tension can be created by *elastic recoil* of the muscle membranes. In this situation a third process also occurs. When a muscle is stretched rapidly, a 'stretch reflex' takes place, which tightens the muscle to protect it. This reflex action is in addition to the normal contraction of the muscle. This is the basis of elastic strength, where rapid actions are used from a stretched position to develop the type of strength and power used in jumping, for example. Additional strength is gained through the combination of muscle contraction, muscle reflex action and elastic recoil. The three processes produce considerably more power than a single isolated slow lift (see chapter 18).

There is also a relationship between speed of movement (velocity) and strength (force) – in fact, there is a trade-off of one for the other *(called the force-velocity trade-off)*. When a very heavy weight is lifted there is a tendency to lift it very slowly with a strong action using all the muscles fibres. A faster movement will develop more speed, but less strength. This is partly because there is less time available for the actin and myosin elements of the muscle to couple.

When training for a particular sporting action it is important that the speed of an exercise closely matches that of the movement to be carried out in the sport. This is because the changes occurring in the muscle, which cause it to become stronger, will be matched (specific) to the speed of the exercise. One of the reasons this occurs is because fast exercises will recruit more of the fast-twitch fibres of a muscle and the slow-twitch fibres will not be as active. This leads to an increase in size of only the fast-twitch fibres, a process known as *preferential hypertrophy*.

THE GROUP ACTION OF MUSCLES

A muscle can only pull; it cannot decide which action to perform. We perform an infinite variety of actions with a finite number of muscles by combining the various actions in different ways. The coordinated action of the various muscles responsible for moving a body part is called the *group action*.

When a muscle pulls to create a movement it is said to be acting as a *prime mover* or agonist. Most muscles can take on this function, depending on the action required and the site of the muscle. The prime mover is often associated with weight training. For example, the biceps muscle of the arm is exercised by performing an arm curl. In this situation, the biceps is the prime mover. In a leg curl, the prime movers are the hamstrings; in a leg extension the prime mover is the quadriceps. In some situations two muscles could create a movement, for example during hip extension on a multihip unit (p. 151). Both the hamstrings and the gluteal muscles can perform this action. The muscle which contributes most to the action is the prime mover, while the muscle which assists in the action is the *assistant mover* or secondary mover.

However, to restrict ourselves to the use of a muscle merely as a mover will greatly reduce the variety of possible exercises and may make our training too restricted. We must look at other types of muscle action and see if these are also relevant to bodytoning.

The muscle which if it contracted would oppose the prime mover is known as the *antagonist*. In the above example we saw that when the biceps contracts to bend the elbow it is acting as a prime mover. To allow this movement to take place the triceps, which would ordinarily straighten the arm, must relax. In this instance the triceps is acting as the antagonist, and its relaxation occurs as a result of an important muscle reflex called *reciprocal innervation*.

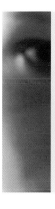

Reciprocal innervation

Reciprocal innervation is especially useful when trying to increase the flexibility of a muscle. For example, if we want to increase the flexibility of the hamstrings, we will get a better stretch by contracting the quadriceps at the same time. This is because the hamstrings in this situation are antagonists to the quadriceps and will therefore relax, allowing us to stretch them that little bit further. For more information on stretching of this type see Norris 1999.

Muscles do not simply create movement; they are also able to stabilise parts of the body or to prevent unwanted movements by acting as 'stabilisers' or 'fixators'. In such cases the muscle will contract to steady or support the bone to which the prime mover is attached.

For example, the deltoid muscle contracts to move the upper arm. Because this muscle is also attached to the shoulder blade (scapula), it would tend to move the blade on the back of the rib cage. To prevent this, muscles running from the spine to the shoulder blade contract, thus acting as stabilisers. The stabilising action can be very important in cases of injury. Although they are only small muscles, if the scapular stabilisers are damaged the whole shoulder mechanism is disrupted and the arm cannot work properly. The importance of stabilising muscles of the spine is covered on p. 68.

Many muscles can perform more than one movement. In the case of the biceps, for example, the muscle can twist the forearm upwards (an action known as supination) as well as flex the elbow. If we just want the biceps to perform one action – i.e. to bend the arm but not twist it – other muscles must contract to stop the twisting movement. These muscles, which eliminate unwanted actions, are acting as *neutralisers*. It is important to understand that the biceps muscle cannot 'decide' which action to perform and which not to perform: a muscle can only pull. If we want to prevent it from bringing about an action, other muscles must come into play as neutralisers.

FURTHER MUSCLE ACTIONS

As well as the standard actions described above, muscles have a number of other obscure functions. These are less important in the context of bodytoning, and so will be discussed only briefly.

HOW MUSCLES WORK

Ballistic contractions

Ballistic actions occur when rapid exercise sequences are performed. Here, the momentum of the moving limb is used to reduce the amount of muscle force required to keep the action going.

For example, when we swing the arm vigorously forwards and backwards when marching or running, muscles contract to propel the arm forwards. Others stop the arm at the end of the movement, and then move it back to its starting position. By using the momentum of the limb in this fashion, energy used during muscle contraction is reduced and the movement is more efficient. Although ballistic actions are not used commonly with weight training, they will be used during a bodytoning workout. Walking on a cross trainer or jogging on a treadmill are both examples of ballistic actions.

Pre-loading

Pre-loading occurs when the antagonist is worked immediately prior to the contraction of the agonist. For example, it has been found that greater force is generated from the quadriceps when the knee is bent before it is straightened. This forms the basis of pre-loading (pre-stretching), a technique used in bodybuilding and powerlifting especially. The additional force created during pre-loading comes from several sources. At slow speeds (holding a weight on the chest prior to a bench press exercise, for example) the laxity or 'crimp' in the muscle tissues is taken up. As a muscle contracts, it must first tighten and take up the slack in the fibres before it can effectively pull against an external resistance. This is a little like giving someone a running start in a race. The processes required for muscle contraction take time to switch on, and by pre-loading the exercise begins when the muscle contraction has already been switched on, so power production is immediate. At fast speeds (a depth jump movement, for example) additional factors are used. Now, elastic recoil of the muscle framework and the protective reflex of the muscle (stretch reflex) provide force in addition to that created by muscle contraction. The result is that additional poundages can be used.

TWO-JOINT MUSCLES

Some muscles have an effect on two joints, they are said to be 'biarticular'. The hamstrings, for example, are able to bend the knee and extend the hip, while rectus femoris on the front of the thigh can flex the hip and extend the knee.

To prevent these muscles from getting too short and thus losing tension, one end will shorten while the other is stretched so that the overall length of the muscle remains the same. Take as an example the walking action. As the hip is extended the upper part of the hamstrings is shortened; at the same time the knee is extended, so the lower part of the hamstrings is stretched. The end result is that the muscle maintains its length and therefore its tension. If the same action were carried out instead by two individual muscles, one would lose tension by overstretching, the other by overshortening. By linking the muscles together, this tension loss is avoided. In addition, the two-joint muscle also gains power through the stretch at one of the joints. In the above example, stretch in the hamstrings through knee extension pre-loads the muscle, providing greater force for the hip extension movement to occur.

TYPES OF MUSCLE CONTRACTION

Imagine that you are performing an arm curl. When you bend your arm and lift the weight your biceps muscle is said to be working concentrically. A concentric action occurs when a muscle is shortening and so reducing the angle made by the bones of the joint. With this type of contraction, the limb is accelerating and building momentum. This is the movement normally associated with weight training; used in isolation, however, concentric contractions can cause imbalances in strength development.

If in the example of the arm curl you hold the weight still, by muscle force alone, the muscle is said to be working isometrically. An isometric contraction is produced when there is no change in the external length of the muscle. This type of contraction is used to sta bilise a joint and hold it locked in one position. It is also very useful after injury to a joint, because the muscle can be kept strong without moving and therefore stressing the joint.

When the weight used in our arm curl is lowered under control, the muscle is lengthening but still producing tension. In such a situation it is said to be acting eccentrically. Eccentric contractions are frequently used to resist gravity, the muscles acting as a 'brake' and decelerating the movement. The tension generated is greater than that produced by other contractions, so more weight can be handled. This feature is used to advantage with 'negative reps' (p. 93).

In the case of the concentric and eccentric muscle actions described above, the speed of movement may vary. As the arm curl is performed, certain parts of the motion can be performed quite quickly, while the part of the movement near the 'sticking point' at the horizontal is likely to be slower. With these two types of contraction the resistance is constant, but the speed of movement will vary depending on how hard you push or pull.

Another type of contraction can occur, during which the speed of movement is kept constant mechanically by constantly changing the resistance. This is called an isokinetic contraction, and is very safe because the resistance can never exceed the strength of the muscle. At the moment, machinery allowing this type of training is very expensive and so is limited to medical and research facilities. However, as the price of the machinery comes down we may well see this apparatus more frequently in the gym.

RANGE OF MOVEMENT

The range of movement (ROM) of a muscle refers to the length of the muscle at any given time. Outer range is from a fully stretched position to the mid-point in the movement. Inner range is from this point to a fully shortened position of the muscle. Mid-range is an area between these two extremes, and is the region in which most everyday movements take place (see Fig. 3.4).

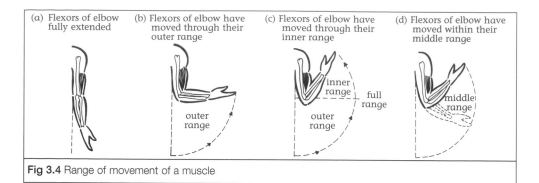

(a) Flexors of elbow fully extended
(b) Flexors of elbow have moved through their outer range
(c) Flexors of elbow have moved through their inner range
(d) Flexors of elbow have moved within their middle range

Fig 3.4 Range of movement of a muscle

A weight training programme should utilise a joint's full range of movement wherever possible. If it does not, stretching exercises must be incorporated into the routine during the cool-down period to prevent the muscles from shortening and becoming inflexible. In certain circumstances limited range exercises are appropriate to restore muscle balance, however. If a muscle has become weak and lengthened due to posture, it has to be shortened as well as strengthened. An example here would be the shoulder retractor muscles which pull the shoulder blades back. If an individual works at a computer and develops a round-shouldered posture, these muscles will be lengthened. To correct this, inner range exercises rather than full range exercises would be chosen to both restrengthen and shorten the muscle back to its optimal length.

BODY MOVEMENT

Standard terminology can be used to describe the movements of the various parts of the body. For example, bending is called flexion; straightening is extension; and straightening past the midpoint so that the joint bends back on itself is hyperextension. Figure 3.5 illustrates the most common actions.

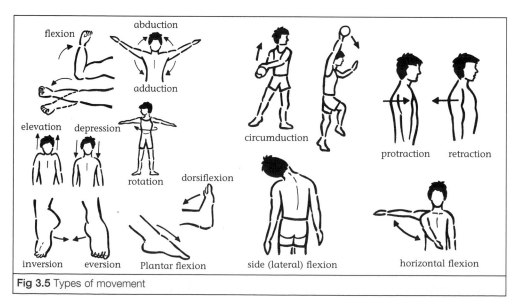

Fig 3.5 Types of movement

HOW MUSCLES BECOME STRONGER

If muscles are exercised at a level similar to their normal daily work, they will not become stronger. When we open a door, or close the boot of the car we are using our arm and shoulder muscles. Although these muscles are being *exercised*, they are not being *trained*. The difference is the amount of challenge that we are offering the muscle. When we lift a barbell, we may be using the same muscles as we do when lifting a teacup for example, but we are working much harder, and challenging these muscles more. This challenge which is over and above the usage of the muscle due to normal daily activity is called *overload*, and a muscle must be overloaded if it is to become stronger, sleeker and more toned.

The amount of work that is used to overload a muscle will be dependent on the size of the weights lifted, the number of times a lift is performed (sets and reps) and the number of training sessions that you perform. In addition, how hard you work and the amount of rest that you take are also determining factors. These variables boil down to exercise *type*, *intensity*, *frequency* and *duration* and are dealt with in chapter 10.

As we get stronger and better toned, the same weights will become less challenging and will therefore not overload the muscle as much as they did when we first started training. This means that our training is now less effective and we have to work harder to regain the same exercise benefits. Making exercise harder in response to strengthening muscle is called *progressing* the exercise. As we train, we should aim to constantly challenge a muscle by using progressive resistance (weights for example). Failure to do this will mean that we maintain our fitness and do not progress further, a stage known as *plateauing*.

STRENGTH CHANGES IN TRAINED MUSCLE

When a muscle is worked, we actually cause microscopic damage to the muscle tissues. Although not serious, this damage stimulates the muscle to regrow stronger and larger, a process called *supercompensation*. For this process to occur, there must be an adequate rest period and sufficient goodness (nutrients) available from food.

The process of tissue breakdown followed by regrowth is similar to that of hard skin build-up on the hands. If you were to take a rough object and rub it into the palm of your hand you would be actually damaging the skin slightly. If you keep doing this for a short period each day for a month or so, you will end up with a patch of hard skin on the palm. Tissue damage has led to supercompensation, just as it will in training. If however instead of rubbing the skin for a short period each day we add all of these periods up and rub continually (without a rest) for three or four hours, supercompensation will not occur. Instead minor tissue damage has become a major injury and the skin has become red and tender. Although in this second case we may have worked as hard (rubbed the skin for the same total amount of time) we have not allowed a rest period for the skin to become stronger and to supercompensate.

This example graphically illustrates the importance of rest to training. Muscles do not grow stronger in the gym, they grow stronger at night in bed! Rest is an essential component of a good training programme, and too little rest will lead to overtraining and exhaustion.

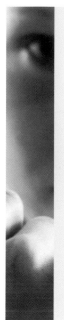

General Adaption Syndrome

The body will react to stress in a specific way, whether that stress is psychological or physical. The process is called the General Adaption Syndrome or GAS (Seyle 1956). Initially there is an *alarm reaction* or 'shock'. This may last for several weeks, and during this time your performance will be impaired and you will probably be quite sore and stiff. Eventually your body begins to adapt to the stress and you enter the *resistance phase*. Your body is changing and making nerve, muscle and chemical improvements which enable it to cope more easily with the stress. This is the process of 'supercompensation'. However, if the stress imposed on the body is too great, or if you fail to allow a sufficient recovery period for the body to adapt, you may enter the *exhaustion phase*. The body becomes stiff and sore again and you lose motivation. Boredom sets in and you have 'overtrained'. Lack of adequate rest, poor diet and too little sleep can all lead to exhaustion.

Two types of changes occur to muscle through training, one called structural, the other functional. The structural changes (called *myogenic*) involve the increase in the amount of muscle protein and the growth of blood vessels into the muscle to make it more effective. In addition there are changes to the chemicals of the muscle which makes the muscle better able to cope with the increased work of training. However, these structural changes do not occur immediately when we start training. Long before that, there are functional changes (called *neurogenic*) which make the muscles work more smoothly and more effectively.

These functional changes involve the electrical charges travelling through the nerve and muscle and the coordination between the muscle fibres, making them contract together as a team rather than in a haphazard fashion. In addition, when you first start training, your body will not allow you to contract your muscles maximally. It does this because the pain of lifting weights is identified as a potential threat which could injure the muscle. Your body stops you contracting your muscles maximally by preventing the nervous impulses getting through to the muscle (a process called *inhibition*). As you train, you begin to realise that the aching and soreness you get is very different from the pain of injury, and your body begins to allow you to work your muscles harder by removing the inhibition on the muscle.

MUSCLE PAIN

Hard muscle training hurts. Whether you are training with weights, gym balls, bands, or in water, if you train hard, you will experience muscle pain. The pain comes broadly from three areas. First, as you contract a muscle and squeeze it tight, the bulging muscle actually flattens the blood vessels travelling through it and effectively cuts off its own blood supply, a process called *ischaemia*. Having no blood both starves the muscle of vital oxygen and also allows chemicals to build up which irritate small nerves within the muscle giving pain, the cause of the *burn*. The build-up of chemicals also causes water to accumulate in the muscle (local swelling) giving a puffed up feeling to the muscle which bodybuilders call the *pump*.

Both the burn and the pump are felt as you train, but you can also get muscle pain two or three days after you finish a workout. This is called Delayed Onset Muscle Soreness (*DOMS*) and results from minor injury to the muscle which allows swelling to gradually build up and a slight increase in muscle contraction (*spasm*). DOMS can be limited by flushing fresh blood through the muscle at the end of your workout. This is the function of a cool-down and is also the reason to have a nice warm shower or even a massage after intense training.

BODY COMPOSITION

Body weight can be a misleading concept. People often talk about being 'overweight' when they really mean over-fat, and about being 'underweight' when they actually mean under-muscled. The total weight of the body is the sum of the weight of a variety of tissues, including bone, muscle, fat, fluids and different types of connective tissue. It can be more conveniently divided into *body fat* and *lean body mass*, or the tissue which remains after the fat has been removed.

Body fat is stored under the skin, around organs, and in bones and nerves. The amount of fat that is desirable can vary, but in general, men should have 10–15 per cent, while in women the amount is slightly higher – around 20–25 per cent. Body fat measurements are useful, because when a person first starts a weight training programme they usually want to tone up and 'lose weight'. In fact, they will probably lose body fat, but their weight may initially increase because toned muscle is denser than untoned muscle.

Many people begin training with the aim of losing fat. Although this may be appropriate in many cases, fat loss must be gradual and controlled. In addition, the *type* of fat which is eaten is also important as well as the *amount*. Certain fats are essential for health, and cutting these out can lead to quite serious health problems (see p. 51).

BODY TYPE

Each of us has a different type of body. Some are fatter; some are thinner; some are more or less muscled. Each individual's body may be classified as one of three extreme body types: endomorphs, mesomorphs and ectomorphs (see Fig. 4.1).

Endomorphs have relatively round physiques and tend to put on and store fat. They have a 'pear drop' appearance, with the abdomen as large or larger than the chest – the typical 'Billy Bunter' character. Mesomorphs have more bone and muscle development. Their bodies are made for strenuous physical activity, and individuals of this type tend to be heavily muscled. The chest is broad, and the shoulders are wider than the waist – the 'Tarzan' type. Ectomorphs have long delicate limbs – the traditional 'bean-poles'.

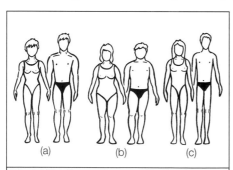

Fig 4.1 The three extremes of body types
(a) mesomorph (b) endomorph
(c) ectomorph

In reality, few people have a physique which falls firmly into one of these categories alone. We are all a mixture between the three extremes. For example, gymnasts and bodybuilders are highly mesomorphic, while distance runners tend to be more ecto-morphic. Swimmers have average scores on all counts, possibly reflecting the fact that these athletes use their own body weight working against water as resistance.

Somatotype rating

By taking height, weight, bone size, limb girth and body fat measurements, an individual can be given a score indicating the proportion of each type of body component present in their physiques. This score, or *somatotype rating*, ranges from 1 to 7, and is presented in the order endomorph/mesomorph/ectomorph. Thus a highly endomorphic individual would score 7/1/1, and a high mesomorph 1/7/1. The somatotype rating can be illustrated graphically so that averages for different sports can be compared (Fig. 4.2).

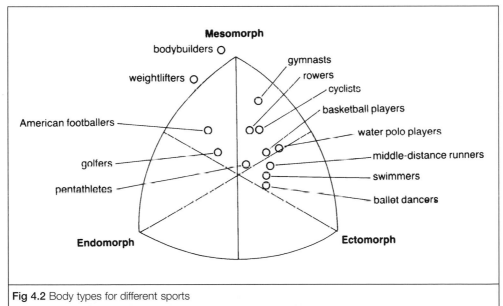

Fig 4.2 Body types for different sports

BODY SYMMETRY

When using weight training to tone and strengthen the body, it is essential that symmetry, or balance of muscular development, is maintained. For example, if an athlete performs more pushing than pulling activities, the muscles in front of the shoulders will be stronger and usually tighter than those at the back. This can create a round-shouldered posture.

Similarly, there must be a balance between quadriceps and hamstring development at the front and back of the thigh. The strength relative to each other of these two muscle groups can be an important determinant of the state of health of the knee. The weaker muscle of the pair can also be more susceptible to injury.

Other important factors regarding the body's symmetry involve the relationship between strength and flexibility. If a muscle is strengthened through weight training, it will become less flexible and possibly more susceptible to injury. To prevent this from occurring, flexibility training must be incorporated into the exercise programme. Likewise, if a muscle is very flexible but is not correspondingly strong, the joint to which it attaches may become unstable.

An important consideration when beginning a weight training programme is the present state of muscle balance in the body. Through our day-to-day activities we tend to favour certain muscles and underuse others. This creates an imbalance state where certain muscles have very high tone and others have very low tone. The high tone muscles (the ones which we use regularly) become tight, and tend to dominate movements – these are our *task* or *movement muscles*. The muscles with low tone which are underused are our *stabiliser muscles*, and they tend to become saggy and lax. Examples of these two muscle categories are shown in Table 4.1. The deeper abdominal muscles and gluteals together with the shoulder blade muscles tend to sag, so individuals who do not exercise and have a sedentary job tend to have saggy bottom muscles, lax abdominals and are often round-shouldered. Because these muscles are not working well enough, the task muscles tighten to try to do all the muscle work. The same individuals often have tight hamstring muscles at the back of the thigh and tight upper shoulder muscles (trapezius) which get painful and develop spasms after a long day at work. When we perform many exercises initially, the high tone task muscles tend to dominate the movement and do all the work while the low tone stabiliser muscles tend not to get worked. To redress the imbalance, the stabilising muscles of the trunk and shoulders must be worked as 'foundation movements'. Only when they are functioning correctly should we begin to perform harder exercises.

Table 4.1 Examples of stabiliser and movement muscles	
Stabiliser	**Movement**
Soleus	Gastrocnemius
Vastus medialis	Deltoid
Gluteus medius	Rectus femoris
Gluteus maximus	Tensor fascia lata
Transversus abdominis	Hamstrings
Internal oblique	Gluteus maximus
Serratus anterior	Rectus abdominis
Lower trapezius	External oblique
	Pectorals

POSTURE

Posture or 'alignment' is something which can be greatly affected by weight training. A generally poor posture can be improved, and specific postural faults corrected. On the negative side, an unbalanced training programme can actually create postural problems. Examples include the unequal arm-muscle development of a poorly trained tennis player, and the round-shouldered barrel chest of an inexperienced bodybuilder.

Posture is maintained both by muscles and by *non-contractile tissues,* for example, ligaments, the joint capsule and fascia.

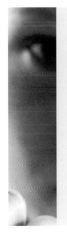

Non-contractile tissue

Non-contractile tissue (NCT) as its name suggests is not able to voluntarily pull (contract) like muscle to create force. It can however create force through its springy elastic recoil. Poor posture which overstretches NCT causes it to become lax and fail to support the body. When ligaments are affected in this way it is termed 'ligamentous laxity' and this is one cause of a joint giving way.

After injury, NCT can be torn and inflamed. When this occurs, scar tissue can be formed within the NCT making it brittle and inflexible. This is one of the causes of postural change and poor alignment following injury.

A good posture is one which places the least possible stress on these structures. Such a posture requires little muscle activity to maintain it, so it is more relaxed and takes less energy to hold. At the same time, joint structures are not overstretched or shortened so much that they cause strain. In both of these cases a good posture is one which is balanced.

Two types of posture are important. Static posture is the body position of a person who is at rest, while dynamic posture is the type of body position that a person takes up when moving. In this text we will limit ourselves to static posture, because an analysis of dynamic posture normally requires complex analysis using video equipment and computers to 'freeze' the action.

Static posture can be described in relation to a posture line or plumb line passing through the centre of the body (Fig. 4.3a). The various body segments all lie on the posture line in a balanced way. Each is placed in a similar fashion to a stack of children's building blocks, with their centre of gravity or 'balance point' on the line (Fig. 4.3b). When the segments

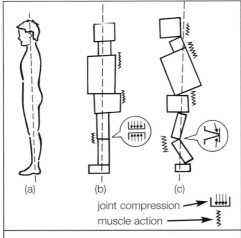

joint compression ⟶
muscle action ⟶

Fig 4.3 Optimal and suboptimal posture

are correctly aligned (the *optimal* posture) they are maintained easily, and so the amount of muscle work required is very small. All that is needed are small flickers of muscle activity to keep the body segments on the posture line. This type of subtle movement is called 'postural sway'. In addition to requiring little muscle work, this posture also loads all the joints evenly. If however one body segment moves away from the posture line (perhaps pulled out of alignment by tight muscles or overly strong muscles) strain is produced. The segment would 'fall off the stack' were it not for extra muscle activity to pull it back. This *sub-optimal* posture therefore requires more muscle effort to maintain it. Additionally, now that the body segments are out of alignment, the joint surfaces are unevenly loaded, increasing the pressure on certain areas possibly causing wear and tear of the joints in time (Fig. 4.3c). The message is clear, the better our posture (closer to the posture line) the less the likelihood of joint and muscle problems.

A number of factors interact to create a person's static posture. Somatotype (see Fig. 4.1) and genetic make-up are both important. So too are strength and flexibility, as well as the way in which you look at yourself – your 'self-image' and your mental state.

On the whole you cannot alter your skeletal structure, so the posture with which you were genetically endowed is permanent (unless you have it surgically altered – children with specific spinal deformities often require a number of complex operations to straighten the spine, for example). Similarly, if you have large or small bones you are stuck with them. You should plan your training programme to take into account your particular body shape.

In the case of both strength and flexibility the important factor is symmetry. An unequal development of either can pull the body out of alignment and so cause postural faults. If a poor posture is being caused by a tight tissue or a weak muscle, exercises can be performed under the direction of a physiotherapist or experienced personal trainer to correct the fault or faults – sometimes with quite startling results.

Finally, a person's mental state must be considered. If someone is depressed, they tend to be more round-shouldered and flat-chested as though the world's problems are pressing them down: a general lack of confidence, particularly in the case of children, can have similar effects. The combination of improved confidence and self-image and the general increase in strength which can result from a bodytoning programme with weights often transforms a teenager's posture so that he or she 'walks tall with pride'.

OPTIMAL POSTURE WHEN WORKING WITH WEIGHTS

The lower part of the back, the *lumbar spine*, should normally be slightly hollow. This curve (the *lumbar lordosis*) is greatly affected by the tilt of the pelvis. The pelvis is balanced like a see-saw on the hip joints, and is controlled by the abdominal, spinal and hip muscles and by the ligaments which surround these areas. The abdominal muscles and the hamstrings will tilt the pelvis backwards and flatten the lower spine, while the hip flexors and spinal extensors will tilt the pelvis forwards and increase the lumbar curve (see Fig. 4.4).

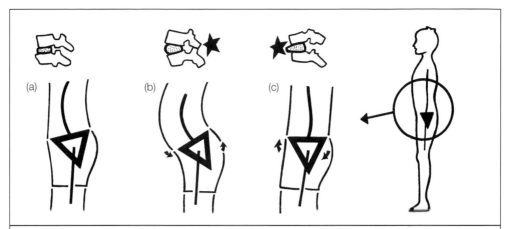

Fig 4.4 (a) Neutral position of the lumbar spine (b) hollow back – facet joints compact; (c) flat back – disc is stressed

These two extremes will stress different areas of the low back. Increasing the curve will compress the small joints (*facet joints*) on the back of the spine while flattening the curve will stress the *spinal discs,* the cushions between the bones of the back (vertebrae). In an optimal posture, the lumbar curve should be midway between these two extremes, so that neither the facet joints nor the discs are overloaded. This midway position is called the *neutral position* and having the spine 'in neutral' or working with the spine in its 'neutral position' when using weights is important to reduce the risk of injury. Exercises such as arm curls and overhead presses for example tend to force the spine out of its neutral position and excessively hollow the low back, increasing the likelihood of injury. Adjusting the foot position to alter body alignment and moving the weight bar closer to the body posture line can correct this (Fig. 4.5).

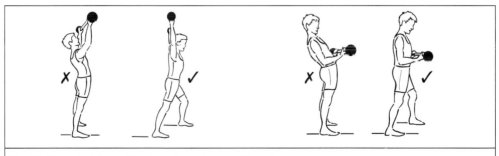

Fig 4.5 Altering body position to reduce stress on the spine

COMMON POSTURAL FAULTS

Lower back

Weak abdominal muscles or tight hip flexors often allow the pelvis to drop and tilt too far, increasing the lumbar curve. This type of posture called *lordotic* is seen particularly in individuals who are overweight. Working on the abdominals and stretching the hip flexors will go some way towards normalising the lumbar curve and can greatly reduce back pain. The abdominal muscles have to be worked within their inner range, that is, at the tightest point in a trunk crunch movement, for example (p. 154). As well as strengthening the abdominal muscles, this type of movement will also help to shorten the overly lengthened muscle.

The lumbar curve can also be too flat, especially after prolonged periods of back pain, or with individuals who spend most of their working day sitting down. Exercise can help to restore the lumbar curve in these cases and work the stiffness loose. A simple exercise can be performed by lying on the floor, keeping the hips down, and pushing up with the arms (see Fig. 1.1). Initially push up onto the forearms and over a period of time the arms can be straightened more and more until the spine bends normally. However, if this movement causes pain the person should perform spinal exercises under the supervision of a physiotherapist.

Head, neck and shoulders

The common fault in this area is a round-shouldered posture (see Fig. 4.6). This has the knock-on effect of allowing the head to protrude too far forwards (poking chin), and cause the upper spine to hump. This humped spinal posture in turn forces the ribs together and restricts chest expansion. To prevent this fault, or to correct it in its early stages, exercises that pull the shoulders back – such as seated rowing – are used. If the problem has been present for some time the chest muscles may have tightened, as may

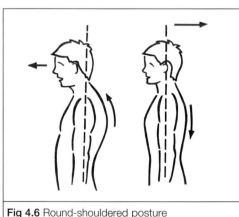

Fig 4.6 Round-shouldered posture

the tissues on the back of the neck. To stretch these structures out, exercises which pull on the chest, such as the 'vertical flye' (pec deck) and 'dumb-bell flye', should be chosen and performed using very light weights. In addition, pulling in the chin will stretch the structures on the back of the neck. Remember that tight structures take time to stretch, so the movements must be performed in a slow, controlled fashion. The aim is to encourage, rather than to force, the movement.

To help prevent these postures in weight training, body alignment must be good in sitting exercises such as seated shoulder press. The head should be held on the posture line and the shoulders gently drawn back. The tummy must be pulled in and the chest opened. A good sitting posture is one in which the individual 'sits tall' rather than slumps.

When viewed from behind, the neck and shoulders can also be seen to be pulled out of alignment. One shoulder is often higher than the other, and the neck may be tilted. These distortions usually arise from muscle imbalances or from tight muscles, tendons and ligaments. If tightness is the cause, gentle stretching should alleviate the condition. Balanced muscle strength can be restored through a carefully designed weight training programme.

Athletes who use only one arm in their sport, such as javelin throwers and tennis players, often suffer from poor alignment in the head, neck and shoulder area. These individuals can use weight training to redress the balance by working the muscles in the gym which are not worked by their sport.

Lower limb

Postural faults in the foot and leg can affect the efficient functioning of the knee joint, and weight training can help to correct some of these faults. If the foot flattens too much (*pronates*) this places an unnatural stress on the foot and knee structures, and will almost certainly cause pain. This can be particularly noticeable when a person performs a squat (see Fig. 4.7). If this is done in bare feet, or in a shoe which is too soft, the foot will flatten excessively along its inner edge. This in turn will cause the shin bones to twist and pull the knees inward into a 'knock-kneed' position. Constant repetition of this action will stress the foot, shin and inner side of the knee. To prevent this, wear good shoes which support the foot and practise good exercise technique. If your foot has a tendency to flatten even when you wear good shoes, an orthotic may be the answer. This is a specially shaped plastic shoe insert which holds your foot in the correct alignment as you train. They are available from most large chemists shops or through your physiotherapist.

A common problem in sport is pain at the front of the knee, beneath the kneecap. One of the causes of this is an imbalance between the different components of the quadriceps muscles. Normally the kneecap travels in a shallow groove on the front of the thigh bone (femur). However, if the inner quadriceps muscle (vastus medialis) is weak, or the outer knee structures are tight, the kneecap can be pulled outwards too far. This unnatural movement can cause the lower edge of the kneecap to rub on the bone beneath, producing inflammation and pain. Management of this condition involves specialised physiotherapy, but one of the mainstays of treatment is to strengthen the inner quadriceps with weight training using a modified leg extension and quarter squat exercise.

In the case of the leg extension movement, very light weights are used and the foot is turned outwards as the leg is straightened. The emphasis is on the *lowering* component of the movement, taking a count of two to lift the weight, one to hold it and five to lower. With the quarter squat action an empty bar is used and the squat action is limited to the first part of the action only, stopping before the knees begin to bend substantially. Leg alignment is crucial, with the knee being placed directly above the foot to avoid a 'knock knee' posture. Again the emphasis is on controlled lowering as before.

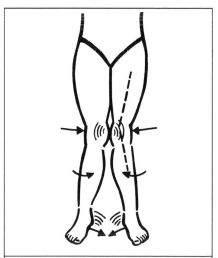

Fig 4.7 Pronation and knock-kneed position when squatting

POSTURAL EXAMINATION

When planning a training programme it is a good idea to work with a partner and to examine each other's posture to see if there are any faults which could be corrected by a well-planned schedule. Standing posture can be assessed from the side and from behind, by comparing parts of the body with a horizontal and vertical line (see Fig. 4.8). Record which side of the body is showing the fault, and compare your chart every six months to determine progress.

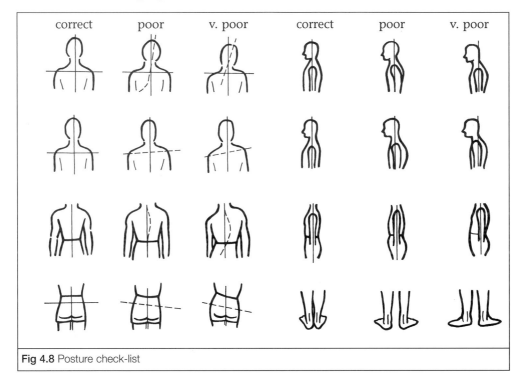

Fig 4.8 Posture check-list

SEX DIFFERENCES AND WEIGHT TRAINING

Sometimes, women hesitate to begin a weight training programme for fear of becoming too muscular. However, scientific studies have shown that both men and women show similar gains in strength relative to their body weight.

Between the two sexes, the main difference in response to weight training is the increase in muscle size (hypertrophy) which usually occurs. Although strength gains in proportion to body weight are similar, changes in muscle girth measurements are substantially less for women than for men. This is mainly due to hormonal differences between the sexes. Pre-adolescence, body muscle size between the sexes are very similar. However, during adolescence testosterone, a powerful tissue-building hormone, is released; men have 20–30 times more of this hormone than women, and therefore put on more muscle mass when they do heavy weight training. In addition, oestrogen levels in women also increase, leading to a deposition of fat around the hips and to breast development.

The precise amounts of hormones will vary between individuals. Some women will have more testosterone than is average, and some men will have less. This is one reason why certain women develop thicker muscles than they would like, and some men find it difficult to build muscle mass, however hard they train. Males who have higher oestrogen levels than average tend to have a softer less defined muscle appearance and carry more body fat. Women who have lower oestrogen levels tend to have less body fat and coarser more defined muscles.

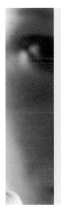

Hormones

During high intensity training hormone concentration in the blood can increase by 10 or 20 times. More hormone is secreted by the various glands, and the rate at which the hormone is removed from the bloodstream by the liver is slower. In addition, hormones act at specific sites (receptors) in the body and the way that hormones attach (bind) to these sites is more effective during exercise. The overall effect of the hormone changes is that the body can more easily tolerate and maintain the high workload of intense exercise.

EXERCISE DURING PREGNANCY

As the female body changes during pregnancy, so the appropriate amount and type of exercise will change. Most women will gain 20–35 lb during pregnancy: their centre of gravity and thus their posture will alter. As the uterus grows out of the pelvic cavity and up into the abdominal cavity the pelvic tilt increases. As a result the centre of gravity of the body moves forwards; and so, to compensate, the lumbar curve is accentuated. Increased breast mass during later pregnancy causes the hump of the upper back (thoracic kyphosis) to get larger, and the head is then held in a protruded position. In addition to these compensations for altered weight distribution, hormones are released to relax the pelvic ligaments and so aid childbirth. However, the effect of the hormones is not just restricted to the pelvic tissues, and all ligaments will become more lax making the joints susceptible to overstretch.

The combination of altered spinal mechanics and relaxation of ligaments often gives rise to pain in the lower back during the later stages of pregnancy. Strength training, provided it is applied with caution, can ease this discomfort by maintaining muscle strength and therefore joint support.

Changes in body composition also occur during pregnancy. There is an increase in fluid retention, metabolic rate, body heat and waste production. These changes are compounded by intense training, which can cause excessive heat gain and reduce the amount of blood flowing to the foetus. Both of these factors reduce the amount of oxygen reaching the child. For these reasons, athletes should train at an intensity slightly below that which they are generally used to, and avoid highly intense exercise altogether during the later stages of pregnancy.

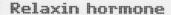

Relaxin hormone

Relaxin hormone is produced from the early stages of pregnancy through to birth. Its function is to produce more movement in the pelvis to provide space for an easier childbirth. It does this by increasing the amount of water in the connective tissue (collagen) fibres within ligaments and tendons making them more elastic. In addition it enables both the abdominal muscles and the pelvic floor muscles to stretch during pregnancy and delivery respectively. Because Relaxin hormone makes connective tissue more elastic, the joints at the front and back of the pelvis (pubic symphasis and sacro iliac joints) become less stable. This is because these are so-called 'fibrous joints' consisting almost entirely of connective tissue. Although the production of Relaxin stops after childbirth, its effects can remain for up to six months after delivery. For this reason, exercises which stress the ligaments in general and especially the pelvic ligaments should be avoided.

Certain positions, particularly lying on the back (supine lying), can interfere with the return of blood to the heart, so exercises such as sit-ups, which require the athlete to remain supine for long periods, should be avoided. Dizziness can be brought on by changing the body position too rapidly, so the athlete should be prepared for this and rest quietly should it occur.

Research has shown that a number of benefits can be reaped from controlled exercise during pregnancy. The duration of labour is less, and labour is generally easier. The likelihood of needing a Caesarean section is reduced, and the average length of hospitalisation is less. Women who exercise regularly also recover more quickly from childbirth. As a general rule, follow the guidelines in Table 4.2.

Table 4.2 Guidelines for bodytoning during pregnancy

- Do not suddenly increase the amount of exercise done.
- Avoid high-risk exercises, such as water skiing, contact sports and skin diving.
- Avoid highly intense, exhausting exercises.
- Do not hold the breath while exercising.
- Always perform a thorough warm-up and cool-down.
- Monitor heart rate and stay well within the recommended limits.
- Drink regularly while exercising.
- Avoid exercises lying on the back on the floor.
- Avoid high-impact activities.
- Do not change position suddenly, as this may cause dizziness.
- Wear supporting/shock-absorbing shoes and choose a bra which gives good breast support.
- Practise good nutrition throughout pregnancy.
- Avoid excessive flexibility exercises because of joint laxity during late-stage pregnancy.

WEIGHT TRAINING FOR CHILDREN

The physical and psychological benefits of weight training make it a desirable pastime for young people, but several precautions must be exercised when training pre-adolescents. In this age-group, fractures can occur across the cartilage end-plate of the bones, and have been reported as a result of overhead weight-lifting activities. Similarly, the soft-tissue injuries which are commonplace in sport can occur during or as a result of weight training. The cause of most injuries is incorrect technique, which places unnatural stresses on the body. Correct technique is therefore of paramount importance in weight training, and especially in youngsters.

Increases in blood pressure with resultant black-out have been noted with the 'valsalva' manoeuvre, in which a deep breath is taken and forcibly held. This technique is not generally to be recommended in the case of inexperienced users. It should never be allowed in the young. In addition, when teaching correct weight training technique to youngsters it is important to ensure that they breathe properly. 'Breathe out on effort' is a good maxim, and it should be enforced from day one.

One of the features of weight training is that it allows an athlete to isolate individual parts of the body and particular actions, and to improve musculature and performance accordingly. This can however create a programme which is too specialised for the young, and pre-adolescent weight training programmes must be planned as part of a general fitness regime so that a proper balance can be maintained. The young require a wide repertoire of skills, which in turn requires a variety of physical training. For them, increases in weight should be seen as considerably less important than a correct technique.

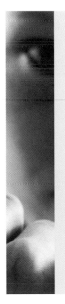

Training and children

Several structural factors are important with respect to training in children. Development of the nervous system will affect both performance and injury potential. Nerves have a waxy coating (the *myelin sheath*) which insulates them and allows nervous impulses to travel faster. This does not completely develop until sexual maturity is reached, so pre-pubescent children cannot be expected to perform fast and skilled actions in the same way as adults. In addition, during the adolescent growth spurt, bone growth occurs faster than both muscle and nerve growth. Imbalances are therefore normal with nerves and muscles becoming relatively tighter as they are stretched over rapidly lengthening bones. The reduction in both general flexibility and muscle balance must be taken into account during programme design.

WEIGHT TRAINING FOR SENIORS

Weight training has traditionally been seen as a sport for young, fit athletes. However, resistance training of all types is used in rehabilitation programmes for hospital patients, so it is easily applied at lower intensities. Older individuals (seniors) can benefit from properly designed and supervised weight training regimes, especially circuit training. Increases in strength, mobility and cardio-pulmonary fitness can be achieved even in later life. As is the case with the young, weight training for seniors should be applied as part of a general fitness programme to provide a good variety of exercise components.

Before starting a weight training programme, a senior should undergo a medical examination, and his or her musculoskeletal system should be assessed by a physio-therapist. This latter precaution is partly to reduce the likelihood of musculoskeletal injury, but also because a number of medical conditions encountered in seniors respond extremely well when a short period of rehabilitation is performed before a general weight training programme is started.

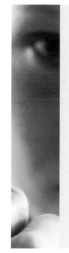

Seniors and weight training

In the early 1980s (Jette and Branch 1981) the lack of muscle strength of seniors was highlighted. In a study of elderly women, 40% of those aged 55–64 years, 45% of those aged 65–75 and 65% of those aged 75–84 years were unable to lift a 10 lb weight. Weight training has been shown to combat these age related strength losses, even in seniors. Individuals aged 87–96 have been shown to increase strength on an eight week weight training programme (Fiatarone *et al.* 1990) and women with an average age of 59 years have been shown to continue to gain strength on a weight programme over a 12-month period (Morganti *et al.* 1995).

BODY COMPOSITION AND FOOD

Fats

A fat consists of a molecule called glycerol with three fatty acid molecules attached, and is more accurately termed a *triglyceride*. The type of fatty acid which is present will determine the type of fat. Each fatty acid is a chain of carbon atoms, with a given number of hydrogen atoms attached at specific points. If all these areas are filled with hydrogen atoms, the fat is said to be *saturated* (the sort normally found in animals) and is usually a solid at room temperature. If fewer hydrogen atoms are present, and the fat has a double connection (bond) between two of its molecules, it is *unsaturated* (the type found in vegetable fats and oils) and is normally a liquid at room temperature. Polyunsaturated fats have more than one double bond and are found in seeds and fish.

Unfortunately, to confuse the matter, an unsaturated fat can be hardened by a process called hydrogenation. It then changes to a 'trans fatty acid', which can be considered the same as a saturated fat. In other words, food may say that it contains vegetable fat, but if this fat has been hydrogenated it is more like animal fat.

Some fat is essential for good health, so to cut all fat from the diet will starve the body of necessary nutrients and make the diet less palatable. In fact, certain fats found in nuts, seeds and oily fish have been designated as 'essential fats' because of their importance to general health. These essential fats are important for things such as joint lubrication, nervous impulses and maintaining membranes within the body.

A general recommendation for improved health is to reduce the total amount of fat in the diet, and at the same time to increase the proportion of this fat which comes from vegetable sources (unsaturated or polyunsaturated fat). Figure 4.9 shows the relative proportions of the various fat types commonly found. Fat should form no more than about 30–35 per cent of the energy intake; of this, saturated fat should make up no more than 10 per cent.

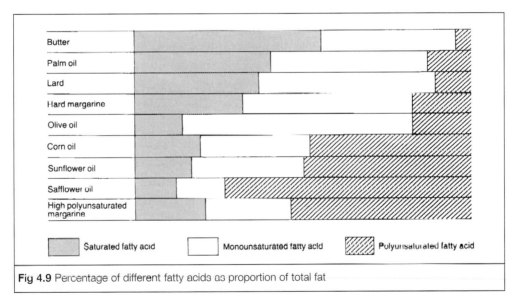

Fig 4.9 Percentage of different fatty acids as proportion of total fat

A note on calories

The energy taken into the body as food and expended during activity is measured in calories. One calorie may be defined as the amount of heat required to raise the temperature of one kilogram of water to 1°C. One kilocalorie or Calorie (with a capital 'C') is the more common measure, and this is equivalent to 4.2 joules, the joule being the other measure of food energy.

Carbohydrate, fat and protein can all be used by the body to produce energy, and so may be measured in Calories. Both carbohydrate and protein produce the same amount of energy, one gram of each producing 4 Calories. Fat is a more concentrated energy source, and one gram of fat can produce 9 Calories, more than double the energy of the other two foods. This is why fat is used as an energy store, and reducing

BODY SHAPE AND COMPOSITION

it from the diet is a good way to lose weight. Another source of energy, and one that is often overlooked, is alcohol. One gram of alcohol produces 8 Calories of energy. Foods are made up of a mixture of nutrients, and so we give each food a total calorific value which reflects the proportional amounts of the various nutrients it contains. This value is useful to those following a calorie-controlled diet in order to lose weight, but does not reflect the quality of the food. This is because high-calorie foods are not necessarily high in vitamins and minerals, and fibre contains virtually no calories at all but is still an important part of the everyday diet.

Energy is expended by the body in two ways. Even when still the body requires a certain amount of 'resting energy' for breathing, heart beat, digestion and other important bodily functions. The amount of energy needed for these processes varies from person to person and depends on many factors, including the size of the body. This resting energy is called the *basal metabolic rate*, and normally uses up about 1200 Calories each day. Energy is also required for voluntary activity, including things such as manual work and exercise. People who have very active jobs or who exercise intensely will burn up more calories than those who tend to be sedentary.

Different sports will burn off calories at different rates. For example, slow jogging may use 120 Calories an hour, while driving a car for an hour needs only 48 Calories. Activities during which all the muscles are worked, such as intense swimming or circuit weight training, can use over 250 Calories in an hour.

Protein

Proteins are often called the 'building blocks' of the body, but they can also be used as an energy supply in cases of extreme need. Proteins are made up of sub-units called *amino acids,* which contain carbon, hydrogen, oxygen and nitrogen (and sometimes sulphur). There are 21 different amino acids which can combine to form a great variety of proteins. While some amino acids can be exchanged for others, there are eight which cannot be made by the body and so are termed 'essential' amino acids. These must be contained in a balanced diet.

The average daily protein requirement is about 0.8–0.9 g per kilogram body weight. More is needed in pregnancy and during the adolescent growth spurt, but for adult athletes – even those engaged in bodybuilding activities – the daily requirement is unlikely to be greater than 1–1.5 g/kg body weight. This is generally provided by the increased amount of food that an athlete consumes, and there is usually no need for protein supplementation. If an excessive amount of protein is eaten it is broken down by the body and the nitrogen portion is excreted in the urine. The amount of nitrogen in the urine can therefore be a good indicator of the amount of protein that an athlete requires.

Both animal and vegetable sources of protein can contain all the essential amino acids. However, in general, vegetable sources do not usually contain all eight essential amino acids, and will be high in some and lower in others. Vegan diets (no meat or animal products) must include a variety of foods to include all the essential amino acids, while vegetarian diets which include eggs and milk products are more easily balanced.

LOSING WEIGHT

When the amount of energy (measured in calories) from food taken into the body equals the amount being expended during exercise and general metabolic processes, an athlete is said to be in 'energy balance'. In this situation he or she will neither gain nor lose weight. If the energy input is greater than the expenditure, the extra energy will be stored as fat. If too little energy is taken in, the body makes up the deficit by drawing on stored energy and burning up fat.

One method of losing weight is simply to eat less. However, in the case of the athlete this has a number of disadvantages. First, it is more difficult to eat a sufficient quantity of nutrients; and second, tissue other than fat is lost, particularly during extreme reduction diets. When a person begins to diet, they lose mainly water. Initially, 70 per cent of the weight loss is water; this reduces to about 20 per cent by the time the person has been dieting for about two weeks. Fat loss speeds up as the diet is continued, changing from 25 per cent of the total weight loss in the early days of a diet to about 70 per cent after two weeks. Protein loss increases from 5 to 15 per cent over the same period.

It is not just the amount of food which is important; the type of food eaten is also significant. High-energy foods (those with a lot of calories, especially fat and alcohol) should be restricted and low calorie equivalents used. The total amount of food may remain the same. It is important not to reduce the intake of carbohydrate-rich foods too much, as these provide the energy for exercise as well as significant amounts of fibre. It is much better to reduce the quantity of high-fat foods and to follow a low-fat/high-carbohydrate diet.

This diet will be more effective if it is complemented by regular bouts of exercise which increase energy expenditure. The body is such an efficient machine that one period of exercise will not burn up many calories. However, the increase in metabolic rate that accompanies exercise will continue for some time after the exercise period has finished, so a half-hour workout will actually continue to burn up calories for three or four hours after the exercise has been completed. Moreover, provided that the exercise is regular, the small number of calories which are used will obviously accumulate so that the long-term effect will be quite dramatic. In this way a person may lose 1–2 lb per week safely, without feeling lethargic. The increase in muscle tone which accompanies the weight loss will add greatly to the overall improvement in physical appearance.

The important foods to restrict are alcohol, fast foods such as chips, and snacks like chocolate and crisps, because these are high in fat. Trim all visible fat and grill rather than fry food. Eat wholegrain bread and cereals, and use starchy foods such as potatoes and pasta, rather than sweet things, to give you energy. Remember also that it is body fat rather than body weight that is important (see p. 38). Someone starting a weight and fitness programme in combination with a diet will initially lose some weight; however, as their muscles become toned and firm, so their density (and therefore their weight) will increase. Although the amount of body fat will be considerably reduced, the change in actual body weight may be less noticeable.

BODY SHAPE AND COMPOSITION

Where a sport requires a particular body weight, practices such as severe fasting and the use of sweat-suits or diuretics are not to be recommended. Loss of weight through these methods is usually the result of glycogen and water loss rather than the elimination of fat. It is unfortunately not possible to replace water or glycogen in sufficient amounts immediately prior to competition, so performance almost always suffers.

GAINING WEIGHT

Weight gain can be achieved through an increase in body fat or in lean body mass or both. In the case of an increase in lean body mass, the changes result almost entirely from enlargement of the muscle fibres through heavy resistance training. Because muscle tissue is composed partially of protein (it is also largely water), some athletes assume that taking additional protein will help to build muscle. This is not always the case. Even the most intensely trained athletes require no more than 1.5–2.5 grams per kilogram body weight, and this amount is easily provided from an increase in food intake. In addition, excess protein which is not used to make muscle will be burnt up as energy or stored as fat. The practice of taking large quantities of milk and eggs to bulk up can in fact be dangerous because it can raise blood-fat levels. When training hard to try to gain muscle, a low protein diet will cause a loss in muscle mass while medium to high protein diets will cause a slow mass increase. However, no greater increase will occur after 2.5 g/kg of protein. Further protein intake will be wasted, being stored as fat rather than converted into muscle.

Athletes often have protein drinks after training, but the timing of consumption is also important. After intense exercise the requirement is for energy food (glycogen) rather than protein. Replenishment of glycogen stores in the body is greatest for the two hour period following exercise so this is the time to refuel with high energy food.

THE MECHANICS OF MOVEMENT ‹

Mechanics is the study of the laws governing movement. Mechanical principles apply not only to machines, such as cars, but also to the human body and to apparatus in the gym. Looking at a few fundamental principles in this area will enable us to understand more fully some of the science behind good training technique.

In all gyms there are mechanical objects such as levers and pulleys, and in your workout you will come across mechanical forces which include friction, inertia and momentum. Let's take a look at the principles which govern all of these factors.

LEVERAGE

Leverage occurs when a rigid bar (the lever) turns on a fixed point (the fulcrum or pivot). Many everyday objects involve the use of levers. The hinges of a door act as a fulcrum, while the door itself is a lever. A can opener is a lever, as is a car jack. Whenever a weight is lifted during weight training, part of your body will act as a lever.

We need to consider two forces when dealing with leverage: *resistance* and *effort*. Effort attempts to create a movement; resistance tries to stop it. In weight training, the weight is the resistance and muscle strength is the effort.

The amount of leverage produced can be calculated by multiplying the resistance by the *horizontal distance* between the resistance and the fulcrum (it is important that the horizontal distance is used, and not simply the distance between a weight and the fulcrum). The further away from the fulcrum a weight is held, the larger the leverage forces produced.

Figure 5.1 shows a simple lever. A resistance of 6 kg is placed 3m away from the fulcrum. Multiplying these together gives a leverage force of 18 units. To balance this out, the effort has to be of the same magnitude. The 9 kg weight has therefore to be placed 2 m from the fulcrum for the lever to balance.

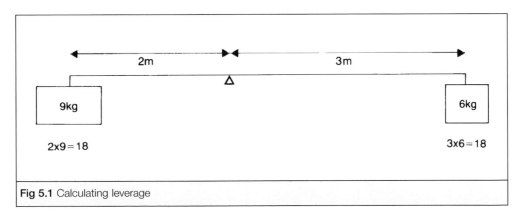

Fig 5.1 Calculating leverage

In the gym we need to be aware of the concept of leverage. A good example of this is offered by the arm curl. As the forearm approaches the half-way point, the leverage is greatest nearest the horizontal. It reduces as the arm nears the vertical. When using free weights, leverage must always be considered; similar exercises performed with the same amount of weight but with different leverages will require very different amounts of effort.

Take as another example the dumb-bell lateral raise (see Fig. 5.2). Here, a dumb-bell is held in the hand and lifted out sideways. Because leverage is calculated using the horizontal distance between the weight and fulcrum, the leverage at the start of the exercise is minimal (the arm is held vertically at the side of the body). As the dumb-bell is raised, the leverage forces increase, reaching a maximum when the arm is held horizontally. Past this point, as the arm is raised above shoulder level, the leverage reduces again and the exercise gets easier.

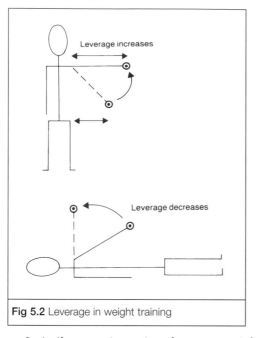

Fig 5.2 Leverage in weight training

A similar exercise, using the same weight but performed lying on the side, exhibits very different leverage characteristics. This time the leverage is greatest at the start of the exercise and reduces as the dumb-bell is lifted towards the vertical. As it moves further into an overhead position the leverage again increases.

Leverage is an important factor when trying to prevent injury to the spine. Because the spine is a long column, leverage forces will increase the amount of force necessary to lift a weight. This force will act close to the fulcrum, which in the case of the spine is the hip. The structure closest to the fulcrum in this case is the lumbar (lower) spine, and this is why low back pain is so common. If a weight is lifted and held close into the chest, the leverage forces are minimal (see Fig. 5.3). If the weight is held at arm's length,

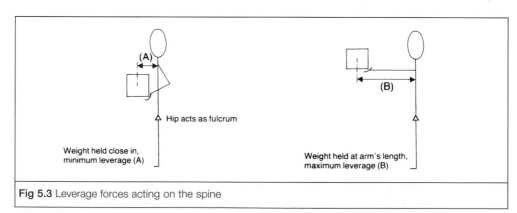

Fig 5.3 Leverage forces acting on the spine

BODYTONING

the leverage forces multiply the effect of the weight by as much as ten times. This will obviously increase the muscular strain on the shoulder, but is also likely to pull the spine forwards, eventually causing back pain.

Various exercises involve potential dangers from leverage, most particularly the squat. When this exercise is performed with the spine upright and vertical a small amount of leverage is created. This is equivalent to the horizontal distance from the fulcrum to the weight, (A) in Figure 5.4. The weight is held on the shoulders, and the fulcrum is the hip; the leverage is therefore minimal because the horizontal distance between these two points is so small. However, if the spine is allowed to flex, the horizontal distance between the weight and the hip increases, (B) in Figure 5.4, and so the leverage force is increased. A squat performed with the spine flexed is therefore potentially much more likely to cause injury to the spine.

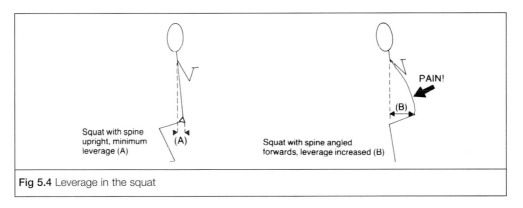

Squat with spine upright, minimum leverage (A)

Squat with spine angled forwards, leverage increased (B)

Fig 5.4 Leverage in the squat

Reducing the length of the lever can make free exercises easier. Take as an example the bilateral straight leg raise (see Fig. 5.5). The leverage is greater when the leg is straight (A) than when the leg is bent (B). Bending the leg thus reduces the strain placed on the spine.

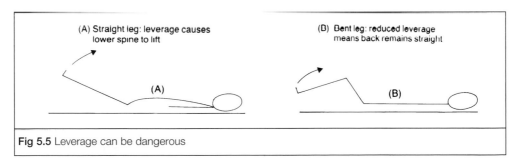

(A) Straight leg: leverage causes lower spine to lift

(B) Bent leg: reduced leverage means back remains straight

Fig 5.5 Leverage can be dangerous

CENTRE OF GRAVITY

The centre of gravity of an object is its balance point, or the point at which all the weight of the object is focused. In an 'even' (symmetrical) object, such as a brick or a weight disc, the centre of gravity is at its centre; in 'uneven' (asymmetrical) objects, such as the human body, the centre of gravity is nearer to the larger, heavier end.

When a person is standing, their centre of gravity lies within the pelvis. This point will change as the body position changes, and, as the centre of gravity is partially determined by the weight of an object, will move when something is carried.

To lift a weight with optimal alignment, the centre of gravity of the weight should be placed near to the posture line of the body. In this position, the weight is easier to balance. Take as an example the squat movement described above. The centre of gravity of the weight bar is in its middle. This point must be placed over the body posture line so that the centre of the weight bar is over the upper spine. If the bar moves to the side, the centre of gravity of the bar is off centre and the bar will tip dangerously to one side (Fig. 5.6)

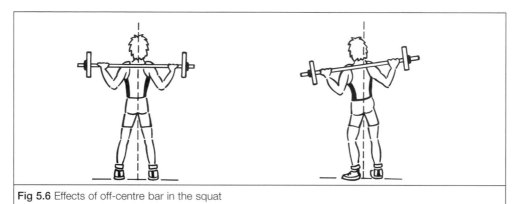

Fig 5.6 Effects of off-centre bar in the squat

STABILITY

Stability is important in the gym primarily for injury prevention. When lifting a weight, an unstable position is a dangerous position, particularly at the end of a workout when fatigue is setting in.

When discussing stability there are two factors to consider. First, the position of the object's *centre of gravity*; and second, the size of the object's *supporting base*. An object with a low centre of gravity and a wide supporting base is likely to be stable.

Take as an example a motorbike. It has narrow wheels and therefore has a small base of support. In addition, the rider sits on the machine and so his centre of gravity is high. In contrast, a racing car has a wide base of support, and the driver sits low in the car rather than on top of it so the centre of gravity is low. The driver's position and the vehicle itself are thus more stable.

The same principles can be applied to situations in the gymnasium. When using exercises above head height, such as shoulder pressing actions, the lifter has a high centre of gravity and so is less stable. Taking a wide stance will help to compensate for this. Similarly, in squatting exercises a wide stance should be used, with the toes turned out to maximise the base of support (Fig. 5.7a).

Widening the base of support in a side-to-side direction will increase the stability to sideways forces. If a person with the feet wide apart sideways is pushed or pulled from the side they will be stable, but not if they are pushed from the front or back. Similarly

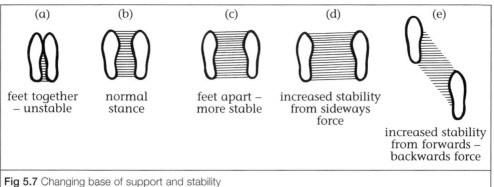

(a) feet together – unstable

(b) normal stance

(c) feet apart – more stable

(d) increased stability from sideways force

(e) increased stability from forwards – backwards force

Fig 5.7 Changing base of support and stability

widening the base of support in a front-to-back direction will increase the stability in this direction. Now the person is stable when pushed from the front or back but not when pushed from the side. The answer is to widen the base of support *in the direction of the movement or force*. So for example a lunge stance (Fig. 5.7e) is appropriate for single arm pulley rows, while a squat stance (Fig. 5.7d) is better for lateral raises.

Many exercises are more stable when performed in the seated position, because the body's centre of gravity is lower. For example, if shoulder exercises are performed seated, the athlete is more stable and less body sway occurs.

To increase stability, then, the base of support must be as wide as possible and the centre of gravity as low as possible. In addition, the centre of gravity should be well within the base of support to allow for minor movements. Adopting these more stable positions when you are first introduced to training will make them second nature in a very short time so that your safety while training will improve accordingly.

MOMENTUM, INERTIA AND FRICTION

These are all forces which work upon the weight that you are lifting, making it harder or easier to move.

Inertia

Inertia is an object's resistance to changes in movement, and is proportional to its weight (mass). The heavier an object is, the more inertia it will have; thus a car is hard to push, and a bicycle relatively easy.

Inertia is important when lifting a heavy weight. It will be difficult to get the weight moving, but once it is on the move less force is needed to keep it going. This fact can be used with very weak muscles in rehabilitation for example. Here, rather than resistance, *assisted movements* can be used. After a knee injury a person may not be able to straighten the leg because of muscle weakness. As the muscle begins to regain strength, initiating leg straightening may be difficult due to inertia of the knee joint itself. If a physiotherapist helps to start the movement, the patient can then use his or her muscles to keep the movement going. Eventually enough strength is built for the patient to move the leg through the whole range of movement themselves.

THE MECHANICS OF MOVEMENT

Friction

Friction is the force which tries to stop one object from sliding over another. Frictional forces are produced by roughness on the surfaces of two opposing objects; if the objects are lubricated (using oil, for example), the friction will be reduced. In weight training, friction is an important factor in the use of pulley wheels. When a weight is being lifted on a pulley, both the weight of the object and the frictional forces between the pulley wheel and cord must be taken into account. Different machines may give very different resistances – even if the same weight is being lifted – if their frictional forces vary.

Friction can also be used as a form of resistance. Some exercise cycles and rowing machines use frictional resistance which may be varied by tightening or loosening a screw handle. This can be simply compression friction of two plates pressed together, or electromagnetic resistance where variation in the electrical current alters the magnetic force pulling against the moving wheel to create friction.

Momentum

Momentum is a combination of how heavy an object is (its *mass*) and how quickly it is moving (its *velocity*). Heavy weights moving quickly will possess a lot of momentum, and can be dangerous if they are not handled correctly.

There is a high risk of a weight with a lot of momentum taking over the movement; instead of being lifted in a controlled fashion it can pull the lifter. This is when injuries can occur. To reduce the effect of momentum, weights should be slowed down and lowered in a controlled fashion at the end of each movement. If this is not done, the momentum still present in the moving limb and weight may tear at a joint and cause injury.

PULLEYS

A pulley is simply a wheel mounted on an axle. In the case of a single fixed pulley the force exerted along the rope is the same at all points (see Fig. 5.8). Fixed pulleys are used to change the direction of a force. For example, a vertical pull in weight training can be changed into a horizontal pull, enabling a rowing action to be performed with an upright weight stack.

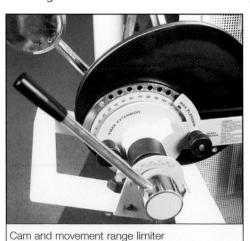
Cam and movement range limiter

Moveable pulleys involve different leverage forces from the standard, fixed type. The edge of the pulley on the trailing rope acts as the fulcrum (see Fig. 5.9), and the resistance comes between the fulcrum and the effort.

The leverage of the effort is twice that of the resistance, and so the actual force exerted to raise the pulley will only be half the amount marked on the weight.

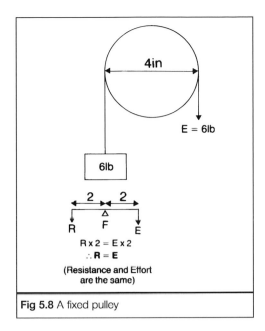

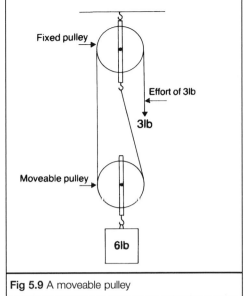

Fig 5.8 A fixed pulley	**Fig 5.9** A moveable pulley

This can be particularly useful in the context of rehabilitation.

Another method of altering the resistance is to change the shape of the pulley, so that it is not round but asymmetrical. This type of pulley is called a 'cam', and is designed to vary the resistance offered to a muscle throughout a movement. In Figure 5.10(A) the resistance arm is slightly larger than that of the effort, and this would be used at limb positions where the muscle is strong. In Figure 5.10(B) the cam has rotated, so that the resistance arm is now considerably shorter and the weight is easier to lift. This cam position should correspond to the weakest part of the movement, or the 'sticking point'.

As a muscle contracts, the resistance which it can overcome will vary depending on a number of factors, for example, limb length, muscle type and length, starting position and leverage. Different cams can therefore be designed for specific parts of the body.

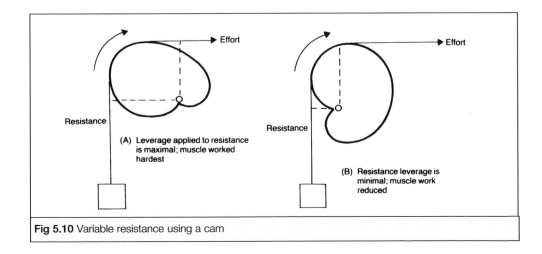

Fig 5.10 Variable resistance using a cam

To increase the strength or tone of a muscle we need to make it work harder than it normally would in everyday life – i.e. to 'overload' it. There are many different ways in which this can be done: weight training, the use of springs and bands, exercising against water and using electric machines are just a few examples.

This section will describe the various types of weight training and resistance apparatus, and discuss the advantages and disadvantages of each.

FREE WEIGHTS

Originally, weight training apparatus consisted of solid *barbells* (used with both hands) and *dumb-bells* (used with one hand). The weights often consisted of solid balls on the end of iron bars, and were used by strong men in circus acts at the turn of the 20th century. As training became more scientific, variable weights were needed; and so removable weight discs and collars were introduced.

WEIGHT TRAINING BARS

A barbell usually has three parts: the bar itself; weight discs; and small collars to secure the weights to the bar. Standard exercise barbells are either adjustable, weights being added to change the total poundage of the bar, or fixed, with weights welded or bolted onto the bar. If the weight is fixed, a separate barbell is used for each 5– or 10–lb weight increment.

For competitive weight lifting, or very heavy training, *Olympic bars* are used. These weigh 20 kg (45 lb), each collar being 2.5 kg (or 5.5 lb). Standard (non-Olympic) barbells are constructed around a steel bar about an inch thick and 5 or 6 feet long. These usually weigh between 25 and 30 lb.

The weight of the bar must be taken into account when calculating how much weight is lifted. For example, if you lifted a bar with a 10 lb weight on each end, you would be lifting not 20 lb, but as much as 50 lb allowing for the bar and collars! A tubular sleeve is often slipped over the bar to allow it to revolve freely without causing friction burns. Cross-hatched grooves or *knurlings* may be cut into the sleeve, or directly onto the bar to provide a more secure grip.

Different-shaped bars are available to facilitate grip, and these are usually exercise specific. For arm curls and triceps extensions an EZ bar may be used. This allows the hand to grip at an angle of 45° to the length of the bar, and both wide and narrow grips can be used. For pulley machines a wide-angled bar is available for the lateral pull down, and a narrow-angled one for the triceps push down. A narrow, square frame may be used for seated rowing (see photo page 6).

Where lighter weights are used for bodytoning, padded bars (powerbars) may be chosen. These are simply different weight solid steel bars encased in resilient foam rubber. They are usually colour coded to reflect their weight, for example, black for heavy (20 lb), purple for medium (15 lb) and yellow for light (10 lb). Because they are padded they are easier to grip and less likely to slip. In addition they are more comfortable to use for the high number of repetitions needed in bodytoning and CV work.

COLLARS

Clamps or collars hold the weight discs in place on the bar. Inner collars are either welded to the bar or form part of a separate barbell sleeve. Outer collars hold the plates onto the bar, preventing them from sliding off during exercise.

Collars come in many shapes and sizes. Some have a threaded key, which is tightened to prevent the collar from slipping; others have a similar arrangement with the screw set flush with the collar and adjusted by an Allen key. The quick-release type are more convenient, however: these are 'spring clips', or keys which tighten in a single movement, and work in a similar way to the locking mechanism on the saddle-stem of a racing bicycle. The bar itself can also be threaded, with the collar screwing directly onto it.

Dumb-bells are simply shorter versions of the barbell, intended for single-handed use. The bars are usually between 10 and 16 in long, and with collars weighing about 5 lb (again, remember to add this to the total weight lifted). A variety of plastic dumb-bells are available, including soft, rubberised versions for bodytoning and CV work. Some are ergonomically shaped to the hand and are more comfortable for endurance work, while others have a strap or band which passes over the back of the hand to aid grip and prevent slippage in repeated activities.

WEIGHT DISCS

There are various types of weight discs. Exercise discs are made of cast iron or steel, and have a hole 1 inch in diameter in the centre. They range in weight from 1.25 lb (0.5 kg) up to about 50 lb (20 or 25 kg). Olympic weight discs are similar in poundage, but have holes of 2 inches to fit the larger Olympic bars.

Some discs are edged with rubber to protect the gymnasium floor, while others are made of solid rubber or special materials such as urethane. The solid-rubber Olympic discs are usually colour coded. Discs for home use may be of plastic-coated concrete; some are even bought as hollow plastic and filled with sand or water at home.

One of the advantages of free weights is their relatively low cost. They can be bought from most sports shops, and the advent of vinyl discs and plastic-coated bars means that a few pounds will now buy the beginner an adequate barbell and set of dumb-bells. Equipped with these, and some instructions on basic weight training exercises, a general programme can be started at home.

The main disadvantages here concern the safety of the user. Weights can be dropped and cause injury, and poor training techniques can cause sprains and pulls.

MULTI-STACK APPARATUS

The increasing interest in fitness since the early 1960s led to the need for safer and more convenient forms of weight training. This has taken the shape of multi-stack weight training apparatus.

Weight stacks

In the case of free weights, discs are added or taken from a bar. With the multi-stack system, the poundage is changed by moving a selector key in a stack of weight blocks. These are usually marked in kilograms, but the weight shown does not necessarily take into account the leverage and friction forces involved, so may not reflect the true resistance being lifted. Some manufacturers use 'split stacks', where the first three or four weights increase in units of 5 kg, and the rest in units of 10. This gives the advantage that there is less of a jump from one weight to the next, making progression of a programme more subtle.

Most weight stacks have guards in front of them to stop users, and particularly children, from trapping their fingers. Even so it is important that users keep their fingers away from the moving weights at all times.

Pin selection

Instead of removable weight discs and collars, multi-stack apparatus uses a removable pin to alter the weight lifted. The pins sometimes have a locking device to stop them working loose. Some manufacturers attach the pin to a slide in front of the weight stack so that it cannot be removed from the machine; in some cases the pins are even magnetic.

ACCOMMODATING OR VARIABLE RESISTANCE

In the case of free weights, the poundage exerted by the weight obviously stays the same throughout the whole movement. However, the force which a muscle can exert does not. This force will change as different leverage forces and muscle properties come into play during the movement.

Ideally, to build a muscle the resistance should be at a maximum throughout the whole range of movement. This is not possible with a free weight, because the heaviest weight which can be lifted will be equal to the weakest point in the range of motion. For example, during an arm curl the leverage is maximal when the forearm is horizontal. At this point the weight will feel heaviest, and so this is the position which will govern the amount of weight which can be lifted. It constitutes the 'sticking point'. At other points in the movement the leverage is less, and so the weight will feel lighter – at these points, then, more weight could be lifted. To make this possible the weight would have to change as it was being used, which obviously cannot happen when the weight is of a fixed amount. However, some multi-stack apparatus uses the principle of *accommodating resistance* to alter the 'weight' as the movement occurs.

 BODYTONING

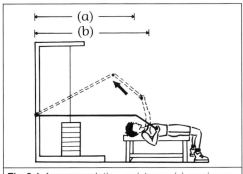

Fig 6.1 Accommodating resistance (a) maximum leverage (b) reduced leverage

The aim of accommodating resistance is therefore to change the weight as the mechanical advantage of the muscle alters. To achieve this, certain exercise stations on multi-gyms have bars which travel through an arc as the weight is lifted. At the bottom position (the beginning of the movement) the lever arm is greatest (6.1 A). As the weight is pushed up, the lever arm reduces and so the resistance to be overcome is greater (Fig. 6.1 B).

CAM-OPERATED MACHINES

Accommodating resistance ensures that the weight lifted is gradually increased in a fairly simple fashion. This feature is extended in the case of cam operated machines (see Fig. 5.10). Here, the shape of the cam is designed to alter the resistance so that it mimics the changes in strength of a particular muscle.

This has advantages in that the overload can be nearer to maximum throughout the range of motion. However, it also means that a separate machine is usually needed for each muscle group. This reduces the variety of exercises available, and increases the expense of providing adequate apparatus.

SPRINGS, BANDS AND TUBING

The lack of portability of free weights and the potential dangers due to dropped equipment led to a parallel development of resistance apparatus based on springs. These were particularly popular for hospital and home use. The spring is a continuous coil of wire with a core through the centre. The spring normally has a 'weight' stamped on it which represents the amount of force required to extend the spring to its maximum. Thus a 5 kg spring requires 5 kg of force to stretch it maximally. The maximum extension will tighten the central cord to prevent overstretching. If the spring is stretched less than to its maximum, less force is required and on some springs the percentage of the maximum is indicated on the cord.

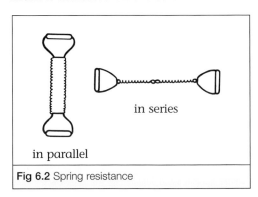

in series

in parallel

Fig 6.2 Spring resistance

Springs may be used for concentric, isometric and eccentric actions and may also be used to *assist* movements, a property used with very weak muscles during hospital rehabilitation. For further resistance springs may be linked together *in parallel*, with two 5 kg springs together requiring a force of 10 kg to stretch them fully (Fig. 6.2). Alternatively springs may be linked one after another or *in series*.

The resistance of the two springs will be the same as that for a single spring (two 5 kg springs in series still giving a resistance of 5 kg) but they will now need to be stretched by twice the length of a single spring to give this full resistance. Springs linked in series may therefore be used where a greater range of motion is required.

A more recent development to springs with very similar properties are rubber resistance bands and tubing. Again these are graded but this time by the density of the rubber used and the bands are colour graded – yellow being very light, red, green and blue being medium and black and silver offering the greatest resistance. Bands and tubing may again be linked in parallel and in series offering the same effects as with springs to increase either resistance or range of motion. An assortment of handles, foot straps and door anchors (used to provide a secure fixation point) are available to increase the variety of exercises available.

THE STABILITY BALL

Stability balls (Swiss gym balls) are now a regular feature of many gyms and exercise classes, and cheap enough for home use. They are normally made of strengthened vinyl and come in a variety of sizes, ranging from 45 cm diameter up to 95 cm. The correct size ball for an individual can be calculated simply by sitting on it. When sitting upright the ball should allow the user to have their feet flat on the floor and the knees and hips at 90°, so that the shin (tibia) is vertical and the thigh (femur) horizontal. Children and shorter clients will obviously require smaller balls, tall individuals will need larger ones. The very large (95 cm) balls are generally used with young children and babies for whole body developmental exercise in hospital physiotherapy departments.

The ball will provide a moveable base of support which will challenge balance especially. They may also be used as resistance or simply to bend the body over for spinal exercise. The ball may be anchored by standing it on a 'collar' to stop it rolling or simply placing it up against a wall. In addition oval stability balls are also used which provide movement in one direction only.

The ball is inflated to offer either a firm or slightly softer resistance. A firmer ball will give a smaller surface both in contact with the floor and to sit on. Slightly deflating the ball makes balance easier as the surface in contact with the floor is larger and the ball offers greater body support.

HYDRAULICS AND PNEUMATICS

Another way of providing resistance is to use hydraulic (fluid) or pneumatic (air) pressure.

With hydraulics, fluid is forced from one chamber into another. The higher the speed of movement, the greater the resistance imposed, so that this type of apparatus does offer the advantage of accommodating resistance. The leverage is changed by moving the distance of attachment of the hydraulic cylinder further away from or closer to the pivot of the machine. Unfortunately, no eccentric component is possible during this type of training: after a bar is pushed up, the opposite (antagonist) muscle group is used to pull the bar down again.

With pneumatics, the resistance is supplied by compressed air created by an electric pump. Resistance is variable, and both concentric and eccentric work is involved.

Both of these types of machine are fairly silent in use; this is seen by some as a disadvantage, because it affects the 'atmosphere' in the gym and reduces the motivation of users. Others see silent operation as a benefit, and claim that the apparatus is safer to use than traditional free weight or multi-stack apparatus.

ELECTROMAGNETIC BRAKING

An electromagnetically braked machine uses the resistance offered by an electromagnet to vary the exercise intensity. The brake may be applied to a lever or a cable system and so unidirectional and multi-directional movements may be used. Most machines of this type only give concentric actions, but some achieve eccentric contractions by the use of electric motors. Because the resistance offered by this type of apparatus results from a change in electric current, users can input data such as age and weight to get a pre-set resistance for their peer group. In addition the unit can be connected to a pulse meter (with the sensor often built into the hand grip of the machine) for pulse rate monitored exercise. This is especially useful where bodytoning and circuit weight training (CWT) are used and also for older or less active individuals.

CARDIOVASCULAR APPARATUS

Cardiovascular (CV) apparatus provides a small resistance which is used over a prolonged time to build CV and local muscle endurance. The machines aim to raise the heart rate gradually and keep it raised during the training period. An electromagnetic brake system is normally linked to a heart rate monitor to vary the resistance depending on the heart rate achieved. Initially there is a warm-up period to gradually raise the heart rate to the training zone. The heart rate in the training zone is normally from 40–80 per cent of the age-related maximum heart rate (see p. 20), the lower rate being chosen for beginners and less fit individuals. When the lower rate is chosen the training period will be longer and conversely when the higher rate is used the training time is shorter.

CV apparatus generally works large muscle groups such as the legs, chest and shoulders to effectively raise the heart rate without inducing local muscle fatigue. The body is positioned in a comfortable starting position which can be maintained for the 20–30 minute period of exercise which is required.

Static cycles, treadmills and rowing machines are perhaps the most familiar CV apparatus in the gym as they have been available for many years. Other apparatus such as recumbent cycles (sitting down), stair climbers (stepper), vertical climbers, and ski machines (cross trainers) are also available. The advantage of the relatively new cross training machines is that they first use a sliding action rather than an up and down motion, thus reducing the effect of gravity on joint loading. Second they normally work the upper and lower body muscles at the same time (as does a rowing machine), giving a more total body exercise.

Core stability is a vital component of any bodytoning programme, and essential before any weight is lifted in a gym. Essentially, core stability is the method by which the spine supports itself, reducing the chance of damage occurring through the rigours of moving, lifting and bending. In most cases when we think of exercising muscles we aim to work a muscle to create movement. For example, if we want to work the biceps muscle which bends the arm, we would probably choose an arm bending action such as a biceps curl.

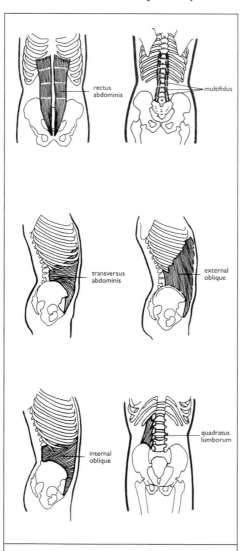

This is using the muscle as a *mover* (see chapter 3). Similarly, when we use a trunk curl action we are using the mover muscle of the trunk which causes flexion (*rectus abdominis*) and when we work on a rotary torso machine we are using the mover muscle which causes powerful rotation (*external oblique*). However, another type of action is performed by muscles which act as *stabilisers*. These muscles do not create movement, but instead *prevent unwanted movements*. An example of this type of action is lifting. When we lift a heavy object, its weight tends to bend the spine and buckle it. To help prevent this and protect the spine, the stabiliser muscles of the trunk come in (see Fig. 7.1). Four important muscles act to stabilise the trunk. The *transversus abdominis* and the *internal oblique* which are deep below the surface of the tummy act as your personal corset, pulling the tummy in tight and making it flat and firm. There are also muscles which are positioned between the individual spinal bones (*vertebrae*). When these work, they hold the spinal bones together, a little like cement holding up a column of bricks. One of these muscles is called *multifidus*, and this is a muscle which a physiotherapist may be particu-

Fig 7.1 The core stability muscles

rectus abdominis

multifidus

transversus abdominis

external oblique

internal oblique

quadratus lumborum

larly concerned with if you consult them for treatment of back pain. Your *quadratus lumborum* muscles deep in and at the side of your spine help to stabilise and protect the back when you hold an object in one hand only.

TECHNIQUES OF CORE STABILITY

The full methods of core stability will not be covered in this text, only an introduction will be given. For a full explanation of core stability together with programmes to develop this important fitness component, see Norris (2001).

In order to work the core stability muscles, rather than moving the spine we use exercises which hold the spine still, and the action we begin with is to tighten the tummy muscles and draw them in, a technique called abdominal hollowing. In addition, we should aim to hold the spine stable in its *neutral position* (see Fig. 4.4). The neutral position is seen when the spine is neither bent forward (flexed) nor hollowed (extended), but midway between the two. In the neutral position the stresses and strains imposed upon the spine are minimised.

ABDOMINAL HOLLOWING IN LYING

Goal To learn the correct muscle control for core stability with the body fully supported.

Technique Lie on your front and focus your attention on your tummy button (*umbilicus*). Slowly draw your tummy button inwards so that you feel your abdomen pulling away from the floor. Hold this contraction for 2–5 seconds, breathing normally, and then relax.

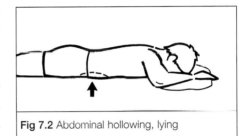

Fig 7.2 Abdominal hollowing, lying

Points to note The action must be restricted to movement of the abdomen alone, do not allow the spine or pelvis to move. Make sure you breath normally throughout the action and do not hold your breath.

ABDOMINAL HOLLOWING IN STANDING

Goal To learn the correct muscle control for core stability training in the upright position.

Technique Stand with your back flat against a wall, and your feet slightly (15–20 cm) forwards. Focus your attention on your tummy button and slowly draw it inwards away from the waistband of your shorts. Hold the contraction for 2–5 seconds breathing normally.

Points to note The movement must be an isolated muscle contraction, do not move the rib cage, spine or pelvis. Make sure that you breath normally throughout the action.

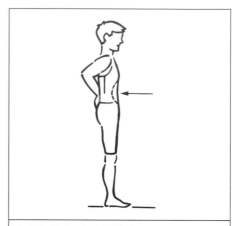
Fig 7.3 Abdominal hollowing, standing

Pelvic floor contraction

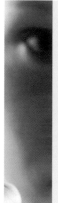

When performing the abdominal hollowing action, it is often easier to get the feeling of the movement by beginning with a *pelvic floor* contraction. To do this, imagine that you are trying to stop yourself passing water (having a wee). The feeling is of drawing up between the legs: for women tightening around the vagina and urethra and for men pulling the testicles upwards. When you have achieved the pelvic floor contraction, allow the muscle tension to spread into your tummy muscles below your tummy button. Feel the contraction tightening and flattening your tummy, creating a space between your tummy and the waistband of your shorts or slacks.

PELVIC TILT

Goal To learn how to increase and reduce the hollow in the lower back (*lumbar lordosis*).

Technique Lie on the floor with your knees bent and your feet flat. Your arms should rest on the floor slightly away from your body. Tighten your abdominal muscles and tilt your pelvis backwards, flattening your back onto the floor. Reverse the action by tightening your back muscles to increase the hollow in the small of your back. Repeat this action three times and then pause midway between back flattening and back hollowing, in the position which feels most comfortable

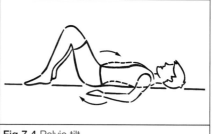
Fig 7.4 Pelvic tilt

for you. This midway point is your *neutral position* and is the position of least stress on the lower back.

Points to note With certain types of posture (see p. 43) the hollow in the small of your back is either increased or reduced. Although you should aim to make this hollow more normal with exercise, initially you may find that one of the two movements is stiffer than the other. If this is the case, encourage the movement, but do not force it. If you get any pain during this exercise, consult a qualified physiotherapist.

HEEL SLIDE

Goal To use core stability to prevent unwanted movement of the pelvis and lower back when bending and straightening the leg.

Technique Lie on the floor with your knees bent and feet flat. Your knees should be 10–15 cm apart. Place your hands on your tummy with your fingers pointing towards your pubis. Tighten your tummy and keep it tight throughout the movement. Slowly straighten one leg, sliding it along the floor, while maintaining the neutral position of your back (see p. 43). Pause and then bend the leg back to the starting position before repeating the movement with the opposite leg.

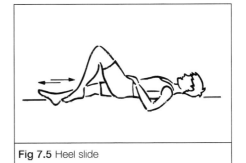

Fig 7.5 Heel slide

Points to note In this action you are trying to maintain the neutral position of your lower back by tightening your tummy muscles and using them to *stabilise* the back. If you find this difficult, modify the exercise by gently flattening the back towards the mat so that it lightly touches the surface of the mat but does not press hard into it (a position called *imprint*). Maintain this imprint position while moving the leg for the first five workouts and then try to maintain the neutral position once more.

LEG LOWERING

Goal To maintain a stable lower back against movement of the whole weight of one leg.

Technique Lie on the floor with your knees bent and then draw the knees up (one at a time) to rest the knees directly above the hips. Gently flatten (imprint) the lower back onto the mat by tightening your tummy muscles and maintain this position throughout the exercise. Lower one leg down onto the mat, keeping the knee bent throughout the movement. When the toe touches the mat draw the leg back up to the starting position and repeat the action with the opposite leg.

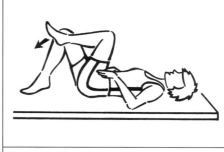

Fig 7.6 Leg lowering

Points to note The foot should be lowered directly downwards, keeping it close to the buttock. Do not allow the leg to straighten, as this increases the leverage effect of the leg and places greater stress on the lower back.

SIDE LYING BODY LIFT

Goal To work the stabilising muscles at the side of the trunk.

Technique Lie on your side on a gym mat with your top foot in front of your bottom; legs straight. Prop yourself up on your underneath arm (either on your forearm or hand depending which is more comfortable).

BODYTONING

Tighten your tummy muscles and keep them tight throughout the action. Lift your hips up so that you form a straight line from your feet, through your hips to your shoulders like a 'plank'. Hold this top position for 3–5 seconds breathing normally and then lower. Reverse the action on the other side of the body.

Points to note   It is the underneath side muscles (*external oblique and quadratus lumborum*) which are working and you should feel them tightening as you lift. Do not allow yourself to sag down or bunch up your shoulders during the movement.

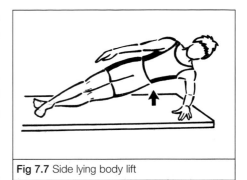

Fig 7.7 Side lying body lift

SPINAL EXTENSION HOLD

Goal   To strengthen and build the endurance of the back extensor muscles.

Technique   Begin lying across a gym bench in the 'press up' position with your upper body free of the bench and your training partner holding your feet firmly. Tighten your tummy muscles and hold them tight while you lift one arm off the floor and reach it forwards in front of you. Hold this position for 3–5 seconds and then lower. Repeat with the other arm. When you have performed this action correctly for 2–3 weeks, you should try to lift both arms up at the same time.

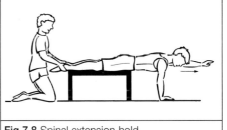

Fig 7.8 Spinal extension hold

Points to note   You must maintain a straight position as you lift your arm. Do not allow your tummy to sag and your back to arch. To help picture this position (*visualise*) imagine you are a puppet with a string at the top of your head. Feel someone pulling this string so that you lengthen your spine horizontally.

Stretching is an important component of any exercise programme. It has a function in both injury prevention and to enhance performance at certain sports. In terms of injury prevention, one of its effects is to reduce *tissue stiffness*, that is, when stretched or moved muscle and ligaments especially are able to stretch more freely. This is a little as though they have changed from being rope-like to being more like elastic bands. Performance in a particular sport will be improved if the *range of motion* (see p. 33) is increased – for example, shoulder flexibility in a swimmer or hip flexibility in a hurdler.

In terms of injury prevention a general flexibility programme is required, but for performance enhancement a more specific programme which accurately mirrors the movements to be used in a sport is needed.

When performing the stretches described below, the end position should be maintained for 20–30 seconds and each movement is repeated 3–5 times. This will give optimal stretching gains, and because the movements are slow and held, there is less likelihood of overstretching. A variety of more specialist stretching techniques are available which rely on muscle reflexes. These are described in detail in Norris (1999).

Because positions are being held for some time, body alignment is important. The starting position should be stable, with little risk of wobbling or falling. If standing positions are used these should be performed near a wall or other support to aid balance. Seated and lying techniques should be performed on a mat, and loose clothing should be worn which will not impede movements.

HAMSTRINGS

Goal To stretch the hamstring muscles using active knee straightening.

Technique Lie on the floor with your left leg straight and your right leg bent at the knee and hip so that the knee lies directly over the hip. Grasp your hands around the back of the bent knee, and use your thigh muscles (*quadriceps*) to pull your leg straight. Hold this position for 10–20 seconds and then release and repeat the action with the other leg.

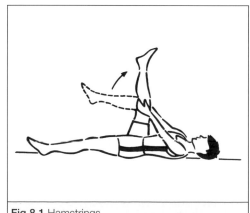

Fig 8.1 Hamstrings

BODYTONING

Points to note   As you straighten the leg there is a tendency to allow the knee to drop downwards. Try to avoid this and keep the knee positioned directly above the hip. The movement also stretches on the main nerve which runs down the back of the leg (the sciatic nerve). If you have had a recent back injury you may feel tingling (pins and needles) or burning during this movement. Perform the action very gently without forcing the movement. If the tingling does not reduce after four or five stretching sessions, consult a qualified physiotherapist for assistance.

RECTUS FEMORIS - STANDING

Goal   To stretch the rectus femoris muscle over the knee and hip simultaneously.

Technique   Stand facing a wall with your left hand touching the wall for support. Bend your right leg and grip your right ankle with your right hand. Tighten your abdominal muscles to maintain the alignment of your lower back and pull your thigh and bent knee backwards.

Points to note   The action must be isolated to the leg moving on the fixed pelvis. If the abdominal muscles are relaxed, your pelvis will tip forwards increasing the hollow in the small of your back. This will give the appearance of being able to pull your leg back further, but the extra movement is an illusion. The increased range of motion is from the spine, not the hip. You can vary the proportion of the movement which occurs at the hip and knee by fastening a towel around our ankle. Gripping on to the towel rather than the foot will relax the stretch

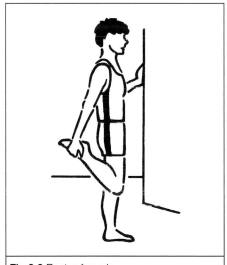

Fig 8.2 Rectus femoris

BODYTONING STRETCHES

over the knee slightly and increase the stretch over the hip. You feel the pull higher up in the thigh as a result.

CALVES

Goal   To stretch the long calf muscle (*gastrocnemius*).

Technique   Begin facing a wall with your feet together, arms straight and hands on the wall. Keep your knees straight and bend your arms to lower your trunk forwards towards the wall. Keep your heels pushed firmly to the ground to feel the stretch along the calf to the back of the knee.

Points to note   Allowing the heel to lift from the ground will release the stretch, and make it less effective. Bending the knee will take the stretch away from the long calf muscle and place it on the short muscle (*soleus*) instead. The result is that you feel the stretch lower down the calf towards the heel.

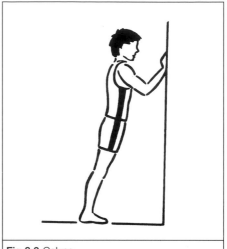

Fig 8.3 Calves

THORACIC SPINE

Goal   To stretch all the surface (*superficial*) tissues covering the back.

Technique   Kneel on all fours and reach your arms in front of you, digging your fingertips into the mat. Sit back on your ankles and feel the stretch over the muscles beneath your arms (*latissimus dorsi*) and over the skin and tissue of your back (*thorocolumbar fascia*).

Points to note   If your place one hand slightly further forward than the other, some

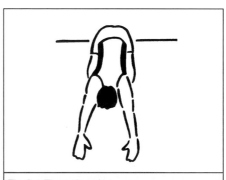

Fig 8.4 Thoracic spine

side (*lateral*) flexion is produced in the spine. Holding onto a low object will introduce a strong pulling force (*traction*) to the shoulders.

HIP FLEXORS

Goal To stretch the deep hip flexor muscles and rectus femons (*iliopsoas*).

Technique Begin kneeling on one knee (half kneeling) with your right leg in front. Tighten your abdominal muscles to maintain the alignment of your lower back. Press your body weight forwards in a lunging action to flex your right knee and pull your leg hip back into extension. Maintain the position for 20–30 seconds and then change legs.

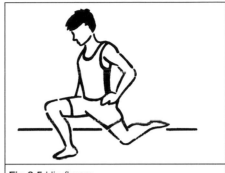
Fig 8.5 Hip flexors

Points to note The effect of the stretch is lost if the abdominal muscles are relaxed and the back is allowed to hollow. The stretch may be more closely focused on the hip itself by pressing the right hand into the buttock of the right hip to encourage greater forward movement.

HIP ADDUCTORS

Goal To stretch the long hip abductors over the hip and knee.

Technique Sit on the floor and open your legs in a scissor action (abduction). Reach your arms backwards and place your hands flat on the ground behind you. Press down to straighten your arms and brace your shoulders, straightening your back as you do so. Force your chest forwards keeping the whole of your spine straight. You should feel your weight transferring from your sitting

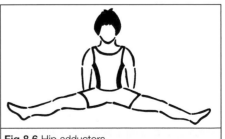
Fig 8.6 Hip adductors

bones (ischial tuberosity) to your groin (pubis) as you press forwards.

Points to note Bending and straightening your ankles will allow you to creep your legs outwards into further abduction. The movement may also be practised sitting in front of a gym machine or wall bar. Hold on to the machine and pull your straight back forwards rather than pushing.

LOWER BACK

Goal To stretch the lower back into extension and restore the lumbar curve (lordosis).

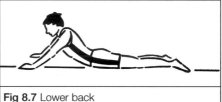

Fig 8.7 Lower back

Technique Lie on the floor on your front with your hands beneath your shoulder in a 'push-up' position. Keep your hips and pelvis on the mat and press with your arms to arch your back. If your back feels very tight just lift up onto your elbows (fig 1.1, page 8).

Points to note If your spine is stiff through prolonged sitting or driving, this action will help to reduce some of the stiffness and back pain. If you have a hollow back posture however (see p. 43), increasing the hollow still further may be painful. Practise the exercise for 10 repetitions. You may notice some soreness and stiffness in the first 3–4 repetitions but this should then work loose. If you experience an increase in pain, STOP and consult a qualified physiotherapist for advice.

SPINAL ROTATION (LYING)

Goal To stretch the spinal rotation muscles (*oblique abdominals*) and open the small joints (*facet joints*) at the side of the spine.

Technique Lie on the floor with your right arm out in a 'T' position. Bend your left leg and twist your trunk to the left, bringing your knee towards the floor. Keep your underneath (right) leg straight to allow you to twist freely. Perform the stretch with the other side of the body.

Points to note If you are unable to take your bent knee fully to the ground, place a rolled towel or cushion beneath it for support at the point of maximum stretch.

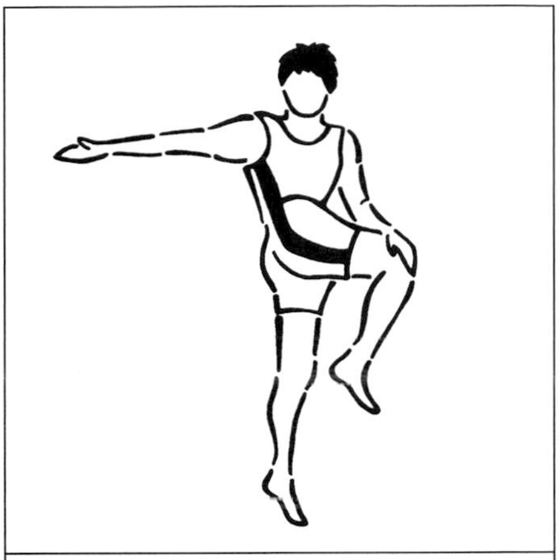

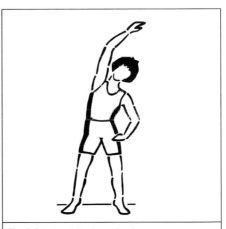

Fig 8.8 Spinal rotation, lying

LATERAL FLEXION OF SPINE

Goal To stretch the side flexor muscles of the trunk (external oblique and quadratus lumborum) and the muscle beneath the arm (latissimus dorsi).

Technique Stand with your feet astride and bend to the right, placing your right hand on your right hip. Reach overhead with your left hand and take it across the top of your head. Supporting your body weight with your right hand, reach your arm over further and increase the side bend motion. Return to the upright position and repeat the movement to the left.

Fig 8.9 Lateral flexion of spine

Points to note If you feel that the side bend stretch is too much for you, you can reduce the intensity of the movement by placing both hands on your hips rather than reaching one arm overhead.

ANTERIOR CHEST AND SHOULDERS

Goal To stretch the muscles on the front of your shoulders (anterior deltoid and pectoralis major).

Technique Stand in front of a doorway with your shoulders and elbows bent to 90°, forearms resting on the doorframe. Lean forwards, pressing your chest through the doorway and forcing your arms backwards slightly.

Points to note This exercise is unsuitable for those with a history of shoulder *dislocation* as it presses the ball of the joint (head of the humerus bone) forwards, the direction in which the joint will normally have dislocated.

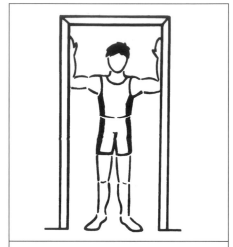

Fig 8.10 Anterior chest and shoulders

UPPER TRAPEZIUS

Goal To stretch the side neck muscles connecting the head to the shoulders (upper trapezius).

Technique Sit on a gym bench and shrug your right shoulder. Tip your head sideways to the left and reach over your head with your left hand. Grasp your head with this hand and use it to keep your head in position. Hold the gym bench with your right hand and pull your right shoulder downwards to feel the stretch at the right-hand side of your neck and inner shoulder.

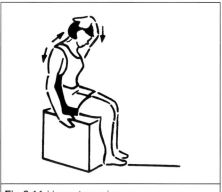

Fig 8.11 Upper trapezius

Points to note Bending the head forwards (flexion) and backwards (extension) will change the muscular emphasis of the stretch slightly.

CARDIOVASCULAR TRAINING 〈

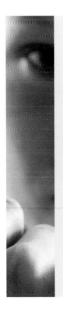

Cardiovascular (CV) training is an essential component of bodytoning, and a significant part of any general exercise programme. We saw in chapter 1 that CV training is important for the condition of the heart, lungs and circulation. This type of training strengthens the heart muscle, expands the lungs and conditions the blood vessels; and these changes are some of the ones which help to protect an individual from heart problems.

Remember that training type (which exercise), intensity (how hard), frequency (how often) and duration (how long) are the four components which will combine to give effective training. To get the benefits of CV exercise, training must average three periods each week, at an intensity of between 70 and 90 per cent of the maximum heart rate for your age group (HRmax). The lower percentage is for beginners, and should be kept going for about 30–40 minutes. Higher intensities will suit more experienced athletes, and need only be carried out for 20–30 minutes.

How much exercise should you do?

The American College of Sports Medicine (ACSM) has made a number of recommendations about the quantity and quality of exercise required to maintain health. To maintain aerobic fitness (stamina) and correct body composition (body fat %) they recommended three to five days training per week at an intensity of 60–90% maximum heart rate (50–85% VO2 Max). This should be carried out for a duration of 15–60 minutes and be continuous and rhythmical in nature (ACSM 1978). To maintain muscle strength tone and density, they recommended the addition of resistance training. This should be carried out for at least one set of 8–12 reps on the major muscles for two days per week (ACSM 1990). Such a programme should involve both machine and free weight exercises, and be progressive (ACSM 2002).

In the gym there are three main ways to use CV training. First, there are the specialised CV machines to be described in this chapter. Second, circuit weight training (CWT) described in chapter 14 can be used, and third most gyms offer a variety of classes, many of which will work the CV system. Any exercise can be used for CV training providing it raises the heart rate and keeps it high for at least 15 minutes.

Before exercising with CV apparatus adjust the machine for comfort and begin with 2–3 minutes gentle activity before gradually increasing the workload.

STATIC CYCLE

Goal To work the CV system with minimal knee loading.

Technique Adjust the cycle for comfort. At the lowest position of the pedal your knee should still be slightly bent (10–15 per cent). The saddle should be comfortable and not dig in, and you should be able to lean forwards on the handle bars with a relatively straight back, not overreaching or cramped up.

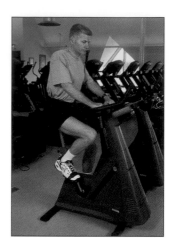

Points to note If you have back pain, rather than leaning forwards on to the handlebars raise them so that you can sit more upright.

RECUMBENT CYCLE

Goal CV training with reduced knee loading and easy access.

Technique Sit on the seat of the cycle adjusting its distance for your leg length. Your legs should remain slightly bent throughout the movement. Grip the seat handles lightly as you pedal.

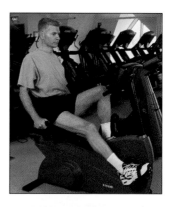

Points to note Stay sitting upright ('sit tall') rather than allowing yourself to slouch.

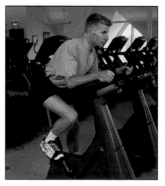

BODYTONING

TREADMILL WALKING

Goal   Gentle CV training taking full body weight through the legs.

Technique   Begin walking slowly on the treadmill to get your balance and gradually increase the speed to a brisk walk. To further increase the training intensity, incline the treadmill.

Points to note   Make sure that the treadmill speed matches your gait.

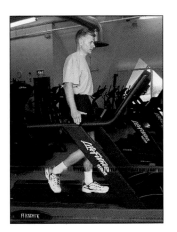

TREADMILL RUNNING

Goal   More intense CV training taking full body weight through the legs.

Technique   Begin walking on a treadmill and gradually increase your speed and that of the treadmill until you are comfortably jogging. To further increase the intensity incline the treadmill.

Points to note   Make sure that the treadmill speed matches your gait. If the treadmill is too slow, you will tend to take short, rapid steps.

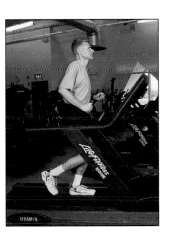

Treadmill speed

Normal walking speed is about 4 mph and normal jogging about 6 mph. If the treadmill is too slow when you are jogging you will take small rapid steps which will unbalance you. To aid balance, first look at a fixed point in the distance rather than at your feet. Begin holding on to the handrails, and as your balance improves let go first with one hand only. As you let go with the other hand keep one finger on the handrail to begin with. For advanced users, slow treadmill walking with the eyes closed is a good proprioceptive exercise. Keep you hands just above the handrails in a 'ready' position throughout the movement however.

STAIR CLIMBER

Goal CV training giving a more intense general leg workout.

Technique Depress one pedal of the machine to its lowest level and step on this with one foot. Bring the other foot up to the higher pedal and hold the handrails of the machine. Begin with slow steps moving through the maximum range of motion. Gradually increase the stepping cadence to suit your fitness level.

Points to note Make sure that your knee passes over the centre of your foot as you step, and avoid a knock knee or bow leg posture.

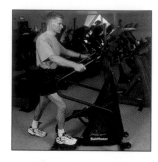
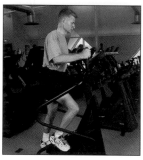

ROWER

Goal CV training with both arm and leg exercise.

Technique Sit on the machine adjusting the foot grips for comfort. Reach forwards and grip the bar, bending at the knee, hip and spine. Pull the bar towards your chest, straighten your legs and angle your trunk backwards at the same time. Reverse the movement to return to the start position.

Points to note The coordination of a smooth rowing action is quite difficult to begin with. Start with just the legs, keeping the arms locked at the elbow, and then use just the arms keeping the legs still. Finally put both actions together and practise a slow precise movement gradually increasing speed as you get more confident. Make sure that you do not lean backwards as you pull (see bottom picture).

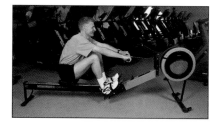
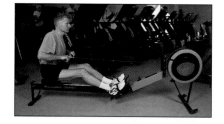
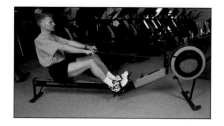

VERTICAL CLIMBER

Goal An intense CV workout using the whole body.

Technique Adjust the pedal height for your leg size and drop one pedal of the machine into its lowest position. Step on to the machine using this low pedal first. Grip the lower arm handle and pull your other foot and hand up to stand square on to the vertical climber unit. Begin the action by pressing down with your higher foot and pulling down with your higher arm. Repeat the movement using a rhythmical climbing action.

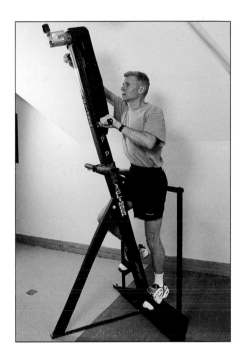

Points to note Because you are using whole body movement in a vertical direction (against gravity) this action is quite intense. It is therefore not suitable for those of very low fitness levels.

CARDIOVASCULAR TRAINING

Goal A whole body CV workout reducing shock on weight bearing joints.

Technique Step on to one pedal of the cross trainer with one foot first, leaving the other foot supported on the side platform of the unit. Hold the handles of the unit and then bring your other foot up on to the second pedal. Begin with slow forwards and backwards actions of the arms and legs, increasing the speed as you gain confidence with the action.

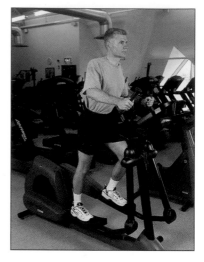

Points to note Try to keep your hips forwards over your feet during this action, and avoid angling the trunk forwards. For advanced users, performing the cross trainer action with the eyes closed provides a useful proprioceptive workout. Reversing the action will change the muscular emphasis of the exercise, increasing the workload on the hamstring muscles. An intensive leg workout can be achieved by holding the static handles and pumping the legs.

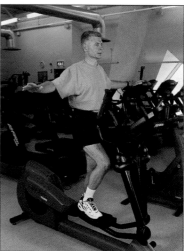

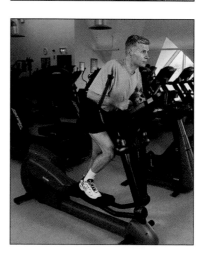

BODYTONING

86

Before exercising, it is important to look at some basic weight training practices and to become familiar with the general terms that will form our 'weight training vocabulary'.

SETS AND REPS

Each time a weight is lifted a *repetition* or 'rep' is performed. A number of reps grouped together is called a *set*. Each set is usually followed by a recovery period.

Traditionally, low numbers of repetitions (4–10) are used to increase strength, while higher numbers (15–25) are used to improve muscle endurance. Numbers of reps in the middle range (12–20) are usually chosen for bodytoning programmes, with fewer reps chosen to target specific problem areas that require extra strength. The combination of reps and sets creates the *training volume*. In general as fitness increases higher training volumes are required to achieve results. When looking at gains in strength and muscle size especially, larger training volumes are needed. For maintenance, lower volumes may be sufficient.

There are no magical combinations of sets and reps which will instantly give the desired results. It is very much up to each individual to find the ideal combination for themselves. This comes with experience, and you must be prepared to change rep/set combinations as you develop. As a general guide for beginners training to improve strength or muscle tone, the weight should be increased when you are able to lift it more than 12–15 times. For best results when strength training, a muscle must be overloaded by working it to fatigue. When you first start training, a specific number of reps may be enough; as you get more experienced, and more able to increase the intensity of your training, you should only stop training when no more can be lifted.

High intensity exercise

Lower numbers of repetitions will enable larger weights to be lifted. This greater percentage of the potential maximum weight works the larger diameter muscle fibres, some of which are only brought on line (recruited) with efforts at 70–80% of maximum. This type of training will achieve the largest gains in muscle size and 3–5 reps may be all that is needed. However, three factors are important when using weights this large. *First*, inexperienced users may not be able to work the muscles hard enough to achieve these results. The

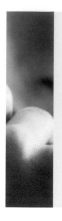

body always aims to protect itself and will not allow muscles to contract maximally when a person first begins training. *Second*, with experienced users there is always a tendency to try to work harder in the belief that the results will be better. However, if adequate recovery is not allowed new muscle tissue cannot grow and overtraining results. As a general rule to avoid overtraining, never begin a workout with soreness from a previous exercise session. *Third*, high intensity exercise is very skilled, and the injury risk is greater. Correct technique is vital at all times if injury is to be avoided.

FREQUENCY, INTENSITY AND DURATION

During resistance training slight damage occurs within the muscle itself. In order to repair itself the muscle needs time, so training should be performed on a particular muscle group every other day in general. Three sessions per week of resistance training is generally sufficient for maximal strength gains. During the rest period between each set, fresh blood is flushed into the muscle to remove metabolic wastes and to replenish the muscle's energy stores.

When working submaximally, a recovery of between 30 and 60 seconds is normally sufficient between sets, but this period will obviously increase when maximal work is performed or as fatigue sets in. At the beginning of a workout you are still fresh, so less rest is needed; by the end, however, rest periods should be increased as you tire. It takes about 3 minutes to 'pay back' most of a muscle's local energy stores, so the muscle will not be fully recovered until this time period has elapsed.

Weight training is a predominantly anaerobic activity (not using oxygen) and therefore it quickly uses up the body's energy stores. The duration of this type of training should usually be between 30 minutes and 1 hour. Longer periods tend to be of lower quality and of little further benefit.

TIMING

When trying to strengthen or tone a muscle using weight training apparatus we must capitalise on all three types of muscle work – concentric, isometric and eccentric. *Concentric* work occurs when a weight is lifted; *isometric* as it is held; and *eccentric* as the weight is lowered under control (see p. 33).

If the exercise is performed too quickly the eccentric phase may be too short and the isometric phase missed out altogether. This sometimes happens when the weight is lifted and then almost 'dropped' by an inexperienced user.

The best way to ensure that all three types of work are done is to lift for a count of two, hold for one and lower for a count of four. In the case of some advanced training

BODYTONING

techniques the lowering period is extended to increase the intensity of work done by the muscle. With postural re-education, the holding time may be increased. Instead of gradually increasing the weight (resistance) lifted, 2 kg to 6 kg to 10 kg for example, the holding time is increased. A typical postural endurance exercise would see very light weight being lifted and held for 10–30 seconds or longer, breathing normally throughout.

ORDER OF EXERCISES

In a basic routine, large muscle groups should be exercised first. The small muscles will be the first to fatigue: because they form the final link in the chain of movement, exercise will stop before the large groups reach exhaustion. For example, both the pectorals and the triceps are exercised during a bench press. However, were you to perform a triceps isolation exercise before the bench press, the triceps would fatigue, thus limiting the number of reps possible on the bench press and therefore the work done by the biceps.

In any workout, the 'priority' muscles – those with which you are particularly concerned – should be worked first. If your primary aim is to build up leg strength, and your secondary aim is to maintain general body tone, then leg exercises should be performed first.

For general fitness training the heart rate should be kept high, but muscles should still be allowed to recover after they have been worked. This is achieved by working the different body areas in turn (arms, legs, trunk, then repeat). In this way, individual muscles recover but overall body activity keeps the heart rate high and thus improves stamina.

TYPE OF EXERCISE

Exercises can be classified broadly as being one of two types: basic (multi-joint) exercises and isolation (single-joint) exercises.

Basic exercises move a number of joints, and so exercise a whole range of muscles. Examples include the bench press, the squat and the shoulder press. Isolation exercises focus on one muscle by trying to restrict the movement to one joint. Examples include dumb-bell flyes, leg extensions and lateral raises. Various basic and isolation exercises are presented in Table 10.1.

SPEED OF MOVEMENT

In any resistance training programme the aim is to overload a muscle by getting it to lift a weight. Fast, jerky actions will increase the weight's momentum. This additional force can then be used to help lift the weight, so that less work is done by the muscle, and ultimately less benefit gained from the training.

WEIGHT TRAINING PRACTICE

Table 10.1 Types of exercise	
Basic exercise	**Isolation exercise**
Squat	Leg extension
Leg press	Leg curl
Lunge	Hip abduction
Bench press	Vertical flye
Shoulder press	Dumb-bell lateral raise
Dips	Triceps extension
Chin-ups	Arm curl

Furthermore, as momentum builds up it becomes more difficult to stop a movement. When fatigue sets in, the increased momentum working at the end of the movement range can overstretch and tear at the joint structures, causing injury. The movement of the weight should therefore be controlled at all times, avoiding any vigorous swinging actions.

Slowing the movement of a weight down not only reduces momentum, but also increases the time over which the weight acts on the body and so increases the training volume. This is a feature used in 'super slow' training described on p. 95.

BREATHING

The general rule is 'breathe out on effort'. As a weight is lifted the muscles bulge. As they do so, the small blood vessels travelling through the muscle are temporarily blocked off, increasing the resistance to the flowing blood. This in turn raises the blood pressure. If at this stage you hold your breath, your blood pressure will increase still further, because the pressure in the lungs compresses large vessels travelling through the chest. If you breathe out, the resultant reduction in pressure inside the chest (intra thoracic pressure) will limit the overall increase in blood pressure.

Another reason to breathe out when you lift a weight is core stability (see p. 68). Tightening the deep abdominal muscles by pulling the tummy button in actually supports the spine by providing your own personal 'muscle corset'. Drawing the abdominal wall inwards as you breath out creates the correct muscle sequence between the deep abdominal muscles and the diaphragm (the muscle sheet inside your chest and beneath your lungs).

Although breathing out on effort is a general rule for safety, there are two occasions on which it will not apply. The first is when you are working for chest expansion, for example, with a pullover or a dumb-bell flye. When performing these exercises you should breathe in.

The second instance concerns the *valsalva manoeuvre*. This is a specialised weight lifting technique, during which the athlete holds his breath and then tries to breathe out against a closed glottis (the 'valve' in the windpipe and throat). The increased intra-thoracic pressure and raised blood pressure give a feeling of strength, and may lessen the likelihood of injury to the spinal discs by contributing to core stability. However, this can cause lightheadedness and therefore should be avoided by all but the most experienced users.

Designing your bodytoning workout

When compiling any weight training programme it is important to have a clear idea of what you are trying to achieve. A bodytoning programme designed to improve general fitness and muscle tone will differ from a workout designed to increase strength. Some individuals may be training to improve their performance at a particular sport, while others may want to lose weight. Training must therefore be adapted accordingly and targeted at specific goals.

BASIC TECHNIQUES

One of the first attempts to change the bodybuilding and weight lifting techniques of the fairground into a science was made with the introduction of the concept of 'progressive resistance exercise'. This was first developed after the Second World War by two doctors, Delorme and Watkins. Although intended at the time to be used in rehabilitation, the techniques have since become the starting point for all types of muscle training.

The method first requires the user to discover the maximum weight which can be lifted ten times – the 10 repetition maximum (10RM). This is established for each exercise by trial and error. The training programme then consists of three sets of 10 repetitions at percentages of this maximal value.

> 1st set: 10 reps at 50% of 10RM
>
> 2nd set: 10 reps at 75% of 10RM
>
> 3rd set: 10 reps at 100% of 10RM

After each set you should rest and allow your breathing rate to return to normal. Early in the training programme this will happen fairly quickly, but as you work through your routine the amount of rest you need after each set will increase. Although the calculation required by this type of training can be time-consuming, it does give the novice user some guidance as to how to progress. It does not take long to get used to the percentages used, and to be able to 'feel' the difference in poundage between the three sets. The programme ensures that you are fully warmed up before you attempt your 100 per cent maximum lift, and so lessens the likelihood of injury. In addition, the initial measurement of the 10RM value and subsequent recording can be used as motivation enabling specific weight goals to be achieved in a certain time period.

PYRAMID TRAINING

In the case of pyramid training, the amount of weight which can be lifted just once (1 repetition maximum or 1RM) is calculated. A percentage of this value is then lifted for each set. The number of repetitions performed in each set is reduced as the weight increases (in contrast to descending sets, see next section).

WEIGHT TRAINING PRACTICE

1st set: 12 reps at 50% 1RM

2nd set: 8 reps at 65% 1RM

3rd set: 6 reps at 75% 1RM, or to fatigue

The weight is still increased, as it is with the Delorme and Watkins regime; this time, however, the number of reps is reduced so that the amount of weight which can be lifted – and therefore the muscle overload – is greater. Enough rest should be taken after each set to allow the breathing rate to return to normal.

DESCENDING SETS (REVERSE PYRAMID)

In this type of training, the pyramid has been turned on its head! You begin with a heavy weight and perform the maximum number of repetitions that you can. You then quickly reduce the weight by moving the pin selector on the machine and perform a few more reps to fatigue. Again you reduce the weight (without any rest) and perform a further set. Generally only 3–4 sets are performed before total muscle fatigue is reached. Descending sets can only be used with machines rather than free weights as the weight change must be rapid enough not to allow a rest period between reps. The combination of heavy and then lighter weights effectively works for both strength and endurance. However, the intensity of the training is such that not all exercises in a programme can be performed to descending sets. Target one or two exercises in a workout only with this type of training and change the exercises between workouts to add variety.

Reps 6–8 to failure (approx 100% of 10RM)

Reps 9–12 to failure (approx 80% of 10RM)

Reps 13–15 to failure (approx 50% of 10RM)

Reps 16–18 to failure (approx 20% of 10RM)

ADVANCED TRAINING TECHNIQUES

If you are training for strength, and have been using weights for some time, you will need to integrate some advanced training techniques into your programme. This is because muscles must be regularly challenged if they are to continue to gain in strength. Eventually, the basic programmes become too easy. Advanced strength training techniques aim to make your muscles work harder, and can be seen as the 'icing on the cake' of your training programme. Try some of the following techniques, and use them to introduce variety into your schedule.

Forced repetitions

Use a training partner to assist you past the 'sticking point' in an exercise. When you get to the point at which you are no longer able to move a weight, your partner can help by just taking the weight slightly on the upwards movement. This should be a slight touch of the bar, in effect momentarily reducing the weight you have to lift. Using this technique as you perform a set of 10 reps, for example, you would complete the first 6 reps fairly easily and then begin to struggle on the next two. The final two reps would be completed as forced reps to maximally work the muscle.

Because your training partner has to grip the bar or machine handle you are using, there are a number of safety considerations. If you are using a cable, your partner must not grip the moving cable itself, or anywhere near the moving weight stack. Instead they should grip at the attachment point of the cable to the handle, well out of the way of moving weights and pulleys. If you are using a bar, they must take care not to knock you off balance as they force the rep. Their grip/touch should be in the centre of the bar. Where your whole body is moving, they must not get in the way and risk being kicked. They should stand at the side. And finally, if they think they should grip around your waist – don't! Many people are ticklish to a sudden grip on this area and the last thing you want when you are pressing out your last reps is to collapse into peels of laughter. On chins and dips, bend your knees and cross your legs so that your partner can grip your shins instead.

Negative work

The eccentric or negative action of a muscle is the most powerful, and is the last to be fatigued. The force produced is greater than that of either concentric or isometric action by about 20 per cent, and so should be the most efficient at building strength. In addition, eccentric work forms the basis for plyometric training (see pp. 190–6). Research has shown that working eccentrically, and therefore lifting more weight than you would be able to during normal training, can give you greater strength gains. However, there is a cost. Muscle soreness results from this type of training, and the use of heavier weights makes you more prone to injury – so take care! It is better to combine all types of muscle work – eccentric, concentric and isometric – during a training session.

To perform negative work during your general exercise programme, lift a weight normally until you feel fatigued and then get a training partner to help you hold it as you lower it under control. Negative reps can also be carried out without assistance for exercises such as dips and chin-ups. With these exercises you simply lift yourself up using your legs and then lower yourself with your arms only.

At the other end of the training scale, negative reps can be used when a muscle is hardly able to work at all after injury. This might occur for example after back pain

WEIGHT TRAINING PRACTICE

where a nerve has been trapped going through the buttock and down the leg. The gluteal muscles are often unable to contract and if a person tries a hip extension movement while lying on their front the gluteals remain lax and the hamstring muscles do all the work. To correct this, the knee is bent to relax the hamstrings and the leg is lifted off the mat. You then try to hold your leg in this position if possible, and as your training partner lowers it back to the ground you try to slow its descent. In this way the muscle is stimulated and will begin to give a flicker of activity. Eventually it will be strong enough to hold the leg off the mat in extension (isometric action) and eventually to lift as well (concentric action).

Exercise	Position of partner ('spotter')
Bench press	Standing at head end of bench
Seated shoulder press	Standing on stool at head end of bench
Lat pull down	Standing behind, holding centre of bar (not cable)
Chins	Standing behind, grip knees (not waist)
Dips	Standing behind, athlete bends knees, grip shin
Machine squat	Standing behind, grip beneath arms (lats)
Arm curl	Standing in front, grip centre of bar
Cable triceps pushdown	Standing at side, grip centre of bar
Trunk curl	Standing at side, press between shoulder blades

Cheating reps

Strict exercise form should usually be encouraged to minimise the risk of injury. Sometimes, however, other muscles can be used to assist the lifter in overcoming the sticking point and continuing to fatigue. This is only appropriate if the movement produced is safely different from the standard form.

For example, if you are performing a biceps curl, and the sticking point occurs as your forearm reaches the horizontal, you can get past this point by rapidly bending and then straightening your legs and using momentum to help lift the weight. This is useful at the end of a set, but if the small movement becomes a large, swinging action of the spine this can be dangerous. Seek assistance from a training partner, or stop.

Shoulders	Arms	Abdominals
Standing barbell shoulder press	Arm curl	Trunk curl
Dip with knees as in 'clean and jerk'	*Dip with knees*	*Use fingers to grip on sides of knees*
	Dips	Cable side bend
	Place one foot on the floor	*Use fingers to grip on to other side of body*

INCREASING THE OVERLOAD ON A MUSCLE

Many of the overload techniques described below are bodybuilding techniques rather than pure bodytoning moves. However, they can still be used in bodytoning to introduce variety, and to move over a sticking point (plateau) in your training. Here, you stop making progress and seem to 'grind to a halt'. This is often due to loss of motivation, and introducing variety is an excellent technique to achieve the same training aim, but from a slightly different direction. Remember there is no single technique or combination of sets and reps which is the holy grail. Certain techniques may suit you at certain times of your training. If they do, use them. But if they don't suit you be willing to say so and change your training accordingly. A technique that is right for one person may not necessarily be right for someone else.

Peak contraction

Uses a final pull as the joint is closing, forcing extra tension on the muscle at full inner range (p. 33), when it is at its shortest. Using an arm curl as an example, the weight is lifted by flexing the arm, but instead of lifting and lowering, the weight is held at the point of maximum arm bend and the muscle is tensed. The hold may be from 2 to 5 seconds. Breath normally, don't hold your breath at this point because isometric activity of this type may increase blood pressure. Keeping breathing will avoid building pressure in the chest which in itself can lead to further blood pressure increases.

Peak contractions work best for exercises where the inner range continues to stress the muscle. In the bench press, for example, the inner range position is when the arms are straight and locked out. At this point however the muscle is resting so peak contractions are not suitable. Exercises such as leg extension, trunk curl, seated rowing and calf raises work well with peak contractions.

Because peak contractions increase tension at full inner range, they can be used as part of a postural re-education programme to shorten a lengthened muscle. For example, if the muscles which brace the shoulders back (retractors) have become lengthened by a prolonged round-shouldered posture, peak contractions using a rowing action would be appropriate to shorten the shoulder retractors again.

WEIGHT TRAINING PRACTICE

Biceps and Triceps (arms)	Gluteals (bum)
Barbell arm curl	Barbell squat
Machine preacher curl (*peak contraction*)	*Dumb-bell lunge*
Dips	Single leg bridge on bench (*peak contraction*)
Dumb-bell tricep kickback (*peak contraction*)	

Super slow training

Increases the training intensity by slowing down the muscle contraction and stressing the muscle over a longer period. Normally the ratio of contraction is a count of two to lift, one to hold and three or four to lower. This may take a total of 1–2 seconds in a normal training programme. With super slow training, this contraction period is extended to 20–30 seconds to further stress the muscle and increase the training volume. Normally super slow training is only used on one or two exercises in a workout and this would usually be on the muscles you are most concerned with. For example, if your major goal is to increase the size of your arm muscles you may use super slow on chins and dips, having performed arm curls and triceps extensions normally. Because the training intensity has been dramatically increased with super slow training, the corresponding rest period following this technique must be lengthened.

Warm-up	5-10 min
Chest press	3 sets
Dumb-bell flye	2 sets
Lat pull down	3 sets
Shoulder press	3 sets
Cable lateral raise (super slow)	1 set
Arm curl	3 sets
Machine chin (super slow)	1 set
Triceps extension	3 sets
Machine dip (super slow)	1 set
Squat	4 sets
Leg extension	3 sets
Calf raise	2 sets
Trunk curl	2 sets
Reverse trunk curl	2 sets
Bent knee fall out (stability)	3 sets
Cool-down and stretch	5 min

Continuous tension

This is really just good training technique emphasised. Many people, in the loud frantic environment of a free weight gym especially, begin to lose good training form. Weights begin to move too fast and momentum builds up. With continuous tension, movement of the weight is slowed down, but not as far as with super slow training. All three muscle contraction types are emphasised, concentric as you lift the weight, isometric as you hold the muscle tight and eccentric as you lower the weight under control.

Rest pause training

When a muscle contracts maximally, the bulging of the muscle fibres cuts off the blood flow through the muscle by temporarily shutting down the capillary bed. The muscle is now working without an oxygen supply (anaerobic). Although this is one method by which we can increase local muscle endurance it also puts an upper limit on the work of the muscle, stopping us from working maximally. If we want to work the whole of the muscle (all the motor units) at an increased intensity we have to rest to allow fresh blood into the muscle. Rest pause training is a method of building on the rest period to increase muscle contraction intensity. With rest pause training an extended rest period is built in after each rep or number of reps, usually no more than three. This increases your ability to lift a heavy weight for a greater number of reps. You would normally perform the first set fairly light as a specific warm-up. The second set would be heavy to fatigue at the end of 8–10 reps. For the third set, a heavier weight is lifted for 2–3 reps and then you rest for 2–5 seconds. Perform another 1–2 reps and rest again for the same period. Keep performing maximum reps with an extended rest period between them until you reach fatigue.

3 reps continuous 100% 10RM

Rest 2–5 seconds

2 reps continuous 120% 10RM

Rest 2–5 seconds

1 rep 130% 10RM

Rest 2–5 seconds

1 rep 100% 10RM

Rest 2–5 seconds

1 rep to failure

REVERSE REPS

We have used both *negative* (eccentric) training and *forced reps*. Now for reverse reps we combine the two. Take as an example a machine bench press action. Working with a training partner, you perform 6 or 7 reps by yourself. As you lower the weight, however, instead of allowing you to lower unhindered, your training partner pushes down lightly on the bar to increase the resistance for 2 more reps. Finally, your partner uses forced reps to help you lift the bar and then they allow you to lower the bar by yourself.

Reverse reps work because the eccentric (lowering) component of muscle contraction can be stronger than the concentric (lifting) component by as much as 20–40 per cent. Lowering the bar by yourself may not work the muscle maximally then but adding that little extra resistance will, by making up the difference between your potential strength and the strength you need to lower the bar under control.

6–7 reps lift and lower normally

2 reps lift normally, partner pushes down on bar as you lower under control

2 reps partner helps you lift bar (forced reps) as you lower the bar by yourself

Single sets to failure

Normally we use multiple sets to allow ourselves a specific warm-up, rehearsing the exact technique required for a lift by using less resistance to begin with. With single sets to failure we drop the initial sets and use a single heavy set. This can only be used by experienced trainers whose technique is faultless and only during the middle of a workout where you are warmed up and not yet fatigued. The advantage of the single set to failure technique is that it cuts down on the number of sets being performed, first saving training time and second avoiding the staleness and boredom that can set in with multiple set programmes. Typically single sets to failure would only be used as one exercise in a group for a single body part. For example when targeting the biceps you may perform chins, followed by two sets of barbell curls and a single set to failure of dumb-bell curls.

Isometric (static) training

We have been emphasising the need to ensure that our training includes all types of muscle work, concentric (lifting), eccentric (lowering) and isometric (holding). However, in the 1960s some research was conducted on isometric training, showing its effectiveness. This led to a number of commercial techniques such as 'dynamic tension' to build muscle in a shorter time. This type of training is now unpopular because later research showed that a whole workout based on isometric training could lead to increases in blood pressure and failed to produce significant training effects on the CV system. However, isometric training if used as a single component in a wider training programme can be used to introduce variety into a workout.

Generally isometric contractions are performed at mid range with the muscle neither completely shortened nor lengthened. As an example, after performing 2 sets of lat pulls, adjust the weight to maximum and pull on the bar without lifting the weight, simply to tense the muscles. Hold the contraction for 5–10 seconds breathing normally (don't hold your breath). Use isometric training for 2 or 3 exercises only in a workout to maintain interest.

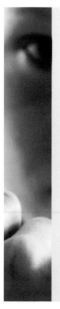

Isometric contractions

Isometric contractions have to be maintained for at least 6 seconds to cause an effective strength gain (Hettinger and Muller 1953). It takes about 4 seconds for a muscle to build up to its maximum tension, but that tension cannot be maintained. After 5 seconds tension has reduced to 75% of maximum, and by 10 seconds the tension drop is by 50% as fatigue gradually sets in. Isometric training (if used on its own) is more effective if practised every day, with alternate day training giving only 80% of the strength increase of daily training (Astrand and Rodahl 1986). Strength gains will be greater at the joint angle that isometric training is carried out, so multiple joint angles should be used. Isometric training has its greatest value in maintaining strength and preventing muscle wastage where an injury has occurred which prevents the joint from moving. It is used widely in hospitals by physiotherapists for this reason.

Multiple sets

Also called 'giant sets' and 'trisets', multiple sets involve choosing three or more sets of exercises for the same body part, with little or no rest between exercises. The advantage of this type of training is that it works the same muscle in several different ways. It introduces variety and avoids boredom. It is difficult to maintain focus and motivation when performing six sets of lateral dumb-bell raises for the shoulders. However to perform three exercises, for example, lateral dumb-bell raises, front raises and lateral cable raises, each for two sets, introduces variety and keeps your interest. In addition, each exercise, although working the deltoid, hits the muscle in a slightly different way. Lateral dumb-bell raises use abduction and medial rotation of the shoulder while lateral cable raises use abduction combined with lateral rotation. Front raises use abduction combined with shoulder flexion to target the anterior (front) part of the deltoid. Perform each exercise for one set without a rest between exercises. Rest between sets and then repeat the movement. For multiple sets to work well, you have to be able to move between equipment quickly and keep the equipment to yourself. It is therefore not suitable for a crowded gym, but better used at off-peak times.

Shoulders	Chest	Back
Lateral dumb-bell raise	Machine chest press	Lateral pull down
Front raise	Dumb-bell flye	Seated rowing
Lateral cable raise	Free weight inclined bench press	Machine back extension

CHANGING THE ORDER OF EXERCISES

Superscts

With this type of training, blood is kept within a particular area of the body (by opening tiny blood vessels or 'capillaries' in the active muscles and closing those within inactive areas) by working opposing muscle groups alternatively. For example, the triceps are worked for one set, then the biceps are worked immediately afterwards. This pattern continues for three sets. This contrasts with circuit weight training where body parts are alternated. The focus between the two techniques is completely different. With supersets the aim is muscle contraction intensity for bodybuilding, while with circuit weight training the aim is bodytoning and CV training.

Chest (bench) press	1 set
Seated row	1 set
Repeat for a total of 3 sets	
Shoulder press	1 set
Lat pull	1 set
Repeat for a total of 3 sets	

Split routines

With a bodytoning programme, we generally aim to train the whole body in each work-out. However, if you are trying to build muscle you may not be able to allow enough time to perform all the exercise sets you need to work the whole body. This may be due to time constraints with your job or other activities or simply motivation. The answer is the split routine, where only certain parts of the body are worked with each training session. This means that you are able to train daily, or even twice a day in some cases. For example, you may choose to work on the arms, chest and shoulders on one day, and the legs, back and trunk the next.

Split routines can last from three to six days, but at least one day a week should be set aside for rest. Examples of split routines used in bodybuilding are shown below.

Alternative 1

Monday–Thursday	Tuesday–Friday
Abdominals (hard)	Abdominals (easy)
Chest	Thighs
Shoulders	Arms
Back	Calves

Alternative 2

Monday–Thursday	Tuesday–Friday
Calves	Abdominals
Chest	Thighs
Shoulders	Back
Triceps	Biceps
Forearms	

Alternative 3

Monday–Thursday	Tuesday–Friday
Abdominals (hard)	Calves
Thighs	Back
Chest	Shoulders
Biceps	Triceps
Forearms	Abdominals (easy)

PRE-EXHAUST TRAINING

When you perform a basic exercise for the large torso muscles such as the chest, shoulders or hips, you are also working smaller limb muscles like those of the arms and thighs. Unfortunately, the smaller muscles will fatigue before the larger ones have been worked maximally. This acts as a limiting factor and stops your training before the large muscles have been worked fully.

To compensate for this it is possible to partially fatigue or 'exhaust' the large muscles by performing an isolation movement. You then continue to train them to full fatigue with the basic movement, a process known as pre-exhaust training.

Take as an example the deltoids of the shoulder. To work these, you would start by performing lateral raises to fatigue; you then progress immediately (without a recovery period) to shoulder pressing. In the first instance the deltoids are working almost in isolation; in the second, they work with the triceps. Although the triceps are smaller muscles than the deltoid and so will normally fatigue first, now both muscles fatigue at the same time as you have partially fatigued (pre-exhausted) the deltoids.

Deltoid (shoulder)	Pectorals (chest)	Gluteals (bum)
Lateral raises	Dumb-bell flye	Hip extension on multhip machine
Shoulder press	Bench press	Squat

STAGGERED SETS

Where large body parts are worked, such as the trunk, a number of exercises are required to work the whole area. With the trunk, for example, exercises are needed for the upper abdominals, lower abdominals, trunk rotators and trunk side flexors. If each of these areas is to be worked for three sets, this is a total of twelve sets! To perform these one after another will be extremely boring. The answer is to use staggered sets. Here you perform a set of abdominal exercises between each exercise for the rest of the body. For example, you may perform 2–3 sets of arm curls followed by a set of abdominals. You then go on to your triceps and come back to the abdominals for a set and then move on to your forearms and back to the abs again. By doing this you achieve two things. First, you split the abdominal exercises up, and second, you are resting the body part which has just been worked while exercising the abdominals. The downside of staggered sets is that you are not able to focus as closely on the abdominal exercises as you keep splitting them up.

Warm-up and stretching	5 mins
CV training	15 mins
Bench press	3 sets
Trunk curl	*1 set*
Lateral pull down	3 sets
Reverse trunk curl	*1 set*

Shoulder press	3 sets
Dumb-bell side bend (light)	*1 set*
Lateral cable raise	3 sets
Trunk rotation	*1 set*
Arm curl	3 sets
Machine crunch	*1 set*
Triceps dip	3 sets
Rotary torso	*1 set*
Squat	3 sets
Cable side bend (heavy)	*1 set*
Calf raise	3 sets
Trunk curl (super slow)	*1 set*
Cool-down	5 mins

PERIODISATION

Training in the same way all the time can lead to boredom and stagnation, with physical development reaching a plateau. The problem is that doing the same workout each week can get very boring. Training becomes a mundane habit and loses its challenge.

The answer is to split the training up to coincide with your individual goals, through the process of *periodisation*. Periodisation came from Russia in the late 1960s. It enables you to concentrate on certain types of training at particular times in the year, allowing one stage of training to progress into another. Four categories are generally used for periodisation.

- Pre-season training.
- Early season training.
- Peak season training.
- Off-season training.

The aim is to cover all the components of fitness, and to build to a peak just before competition or a specific goal, with the overall periodisation programme usually lasting a year. This year-long period is called a *macrocycle* (Fig. 10.1).

Macrocycle																				
Mesocycle 1				Mesocycle 2					Mesocycle 3					Mesocycle 4						
1	2	3	4	1	2	3	4	5	1	2	3	4	5	1	2	3	4	5	6	
	microcycles				microcycles					microcycles					microcycles					
Pre-season				Early season					Peak season					Off-season						

Fig 10.1 Categories of periodisation

The first phase is the preparatory phase, divided into pre-season and early season training. Pre-season training lasts for about four months; early season training for about one month. As an athlete approaches his/her peak season, more skill training and sport-specific work is included. During the peak or competitive season, training will be designed to maintain the particular fitness and skill needed for competition.

Off-season training acts as a recovery period, psychologically refreshing the athlete and allowing the body to slow down after the intense demands of competition. The timing of this period will depend on the type of sport. During off-season training moderate activity should be maintained so that the progress made in the other periods is not lost. Each of these four periods, being divisions of the year-long macrocycle is known as a *mesocycle*.

Although this type of training was designed originally for competitive athletes, benefits can still be obtained by fitness enthusiasts. For example, the casual tennis player can concentrate on weight training in his or her pre-season training, in order to build up a foundation of strength. Fitness training can be brought in during early training, and skill training introduced. Skill training comes to the fore during the peak season, while strength training is usually dropped.

Tennis should not be played during the off-season period so that the player has a psychological break. Instead, light weight training begins again in preparation for the heavy strength training of the pre-season cycle.

The four mesocycle periods can again be divided into typically week-long units called *microcycles*. The microcycle is used to plan your individual workouts in the gym.

PERIODISATION FOR BODYTONING

The type and intensity of training that you use over your year-long mesocycle will change (Fig. 10.2). To begin with you should aim to use light weights and low training

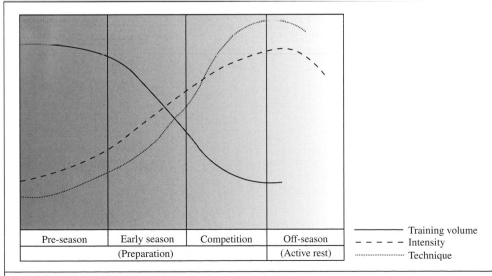

Pre-season	Early season	Competition	Off-season
(Preparation)			(Active rest)

——— Training volume
– – – – Intensity
·············· Technique

Fig 10.2 Periodisation for bodytoning

WEIGHT TRAINING PRACTICE

103

intensities. As your fitness and bodytone increases you can use fewer reps so that your training volume reduces, but higher weights and perhaps some of the advanced techniques designed to overload your muscles. Your training intensity is increasing as your skill (technique) of performing the weight training exercises improves.

To use periodisation, first arm yourself with a year-long wall planner! Mark on it the date of some special event such as a holiday, or sports competition for example, and decide what you want to achieve by this date. This is what you will work up to, and the wall planner represents your personal mesocycle. Lets imagine that you simply want to lose some weight and tone up to look good on the beach for your summer holiday, so we will start before in the autumn aiming to finish next summer.

Next, divide the wall planner into four periods or mesocycles. The first takes in the autumn months up to Christmas. The second is the new year into spring. The third will be late spring and through the summer up to your holiday. The final period consists of the weeks of the holiday itself – you are not going to work out then, so this is your recovery or rest period.

You want to lose weight and that takes time so we will begin the first mesocycle with intense CV training, say 20–30 minutes of medium intensity work on the bikes and cross trainers in the gym. We will also use light circuit weight training to burn calories and tone up. By the next mesocycle, after Christmas, you should be feeling the benefits: a few pounds lost, looser clothing and increased muscle tone. We will continue with the CV work, but increase the intensity so you can now only use 20 minutes of harder exercise. The weight training will become more structured with the aim of toning the hips and thighs and flattening your stomach. Because you are training more intensely you must watch your diet and not cut down on food intake too much. Make sure that you are having plenty of high quality food.

The third mesocycle reduces size of the weights used and simply maintains the size and tone of your muscles. At the same time you increase the amount of CV work to maintain your fitness and keep burning fat. Couple this with full range exercises and stretching rather than bodybuilding exercises to ensure that you get a lean (linear) physique rather than one which is bulky and muscley.

MOTIVATION AND GOAL SETTING

Bodytoning can become quite repetitive and even boring unless you plan your training well. One of the first things to do is to create a training environment which *motivates* you individually. Some people love noisy hardworking gyms with lots of shouting, loud music and clanging free weights. For others this is just hell! Take time to decide what you want from your training environment. You might want to join a gym — find the right one for you. Perhaps you just want to train at the local sports centre with your friend. You may even want to put some simple weight training gear in a room at home. It really doesn't matter as long as it is right for you.

Try using music that you like and choose clothing that you are comfortable in and happy with. Don't wear tight lycra simply because others do. If you hate it, choose loose fitting comfortable clothes instead. It is more important for you to be happy with yourself than to conform with others.

Training with someone is generally useful. This may be a training partner or simply making sure that you go to the gym at the same time to meet people you are familiar with. Another option is to use a personal trainer occasionally. They will be able to motivate you and teach you correct training technique at the same time.

It often helps to be able to see how you will succeed and to be able to imagine or visualise the results you hope to achieve. A personal trainer will often be able to tell you of clients they have who have gone through similar problems and how they achieved results. Knowing that someone has been through the same things that you are now going through can be a tremendous comfort.

Goal setting is a method of maintaining motivation by giving yourself specific aims and objectives as markers of your improvement. A simple mnemonic SMART is often used to aid goal setting, it stands for Specific, Measurable, Agreed, Realistic and Timed.

A goal must be SPECIFIC. What exactly are you hoping to achieve with your bodytoning? Perhaps it is increased fitness, or weight loss or building muscle? Whatever your aims are, take time to describe them to yourself and write them down. How much weight do you want to lose? If you are aiming for fitness, begin with a pulse monitored fitness test. What heart rate do you hope to achieve? If you are building muscle, measure the girth of the limb you want to increase in size, and then ask yourself how much size you want to add. Writing down your specific requirements will enable you to monitor your progress.

In order to know if you are achieving your goals, they must be MEASURABLE. Recording your weight or body measurements enables you to measure your progress. Record this weekly on a chart or training log so that you can see your progress. Don't measure yourself every day because progress will not be that rapid. Have both short-term and long-term goals. Your long-term goal may well be to change from a size 16 to a size 12 but this will not come overnight. Short-term goals are the stepping stones to your final destination. They might be weight loss, girth changes or body fat measures but you will see them achieved gradually and be motivated to continue your training.

Successful training is about commitment, so goals have to be AGREED. Write them down – what do you want to achieve and by when? Discuss them with a friend or training partner or one of the gym instructors. The act of involving someone else places a positive pressure on you to achieve success. This is important when you least want to train and are having an off day. Knowing that you have agreed your goals with someone makes you 'go the extra mile' rather than opting out. If you are training with someone try to motivate them as well. They will also have off days and will need your help as much as you need theirs.

It is easy to say what you want from a training programme when you begin. We would all like to look like the magazine models as soon as possible, but be REALISTIC. What are you likely to be able to achieve? Look at others you aspire to – how long has it taken them to achieve their goals? By being realistic you are likely to achieve your goals and stay motivated. If your goals are unrealistic and too hard to achieve you may well lose motivation and 'fall by the wayside' giving up training.

Finally, ask yourself when you want to achieve your goals. Asking for goals which are open-ended such as 'I want to lose 7 lb weight' or 'I want to build 1 inch of muscle' allows you to take as long as you like to achieve these aims. Again, you are likely to lose motivation along the way, unless you TIME your goals. Setting a deadline will help you to maintain your motivation. Goals should be divided into major and minor units. The major goal may have a timescale of a year for example. You may want to lose a certain number of dress sizes by your next holiday or you may want to achieve a certain fitness level to enter a fun run or half marathon. Although timed, these goals are your ultimate aim and seem a very long way off. For this reason, introduce a number of other minor goals at monthly and weekly intervals to act as the stepping stones towards your final deadline. It is a lot easier to focus your attention (and your motivation) on a goal at the end of the week or month than one twelve months away.

BODYTONING

BEFORE WE START

Before we begin the chapters on weight training exercises, let's first recap on the general techniques of weight training practice that we covered in chapter 1. Before using weights, we need to perform a warm-up which is intense enough to cause mild sweating and takes all the major muscles and joints through their full comfortable range of motion. Look again at Table 1.1 dealing with safety aspects in the gym, and familiarise yourself with these points.

As we go to perform an exercise the machine must be adjusted to suit the user. This may involve changing the seat height and other pads such as back supports, leg rollers and arm pads. If you are using a machine for the first time ask your instructor to explain its working thoroughly.

When changing weights keep your fingers away from moving weight stacks, pulleys and cables. Use a weight which is appropriate, rather than trying to mimic what someone else is doing. Remember the old adage 'never sacrifice technique for weight'. The way you perform an exercise (technique), and the position of your body (alignment) are both paramount in weight training practice.

Table 11.1 Points to note before you use weight training apparatus	
Point	**Explanation**
Warm up	Warm up sufficiently to produce mild sweating, and to take each major joint and muscle through their full comfortable range of motion. The first set of any exercise can also be light to act as a warm-up and rehearse the individual technique of that exercise.
Adjust the machine	Adjust the machine to suit your body size. This may include seat height, backpad and rollers.
Breathe out with effort	Exhale as the weight lifts. The bar may be pushed or pulled.
Work within your limits	Do not try to mimic what others are doing. An exercise should feel safely challenging, but you should always feel in control.
Don't sacrifice technique for weight	If your technique degrades, stop, reduce the weight and then resume the exercise.
Watch your body alignment	Make sure that you sit or stand tall, lengthening your spine. When you practise a leg exercise, make sure that your knee passes over the centre of your foot as it bends. Avoid knock knee and bow leg positions.

In general you should breathe out (exhale) with effort. Practically this means breathing in (inhaling), and exhaling as the weight moves upwards. There are two points here, first, be careful that you do not take so many deep breaths that you go dizzy (hyperventilate). Second, although the weight is moving upwards the bar may be moving downwards (lat pull down, for example) if the aim of an exercise is to pull rather than push. Take a look at Table 11.1 before you try any of the exercises.

UPPER LIMB WEIGHT TRAINING EXERCISES

The major muscles of the shoulder, chest and arms can be worked in isolation or together with many of the exercises given here (Fig 11.1 A and B). The major chest muscles (*pectorals*) act in a pressing action, rounding the shoulders, while the upper back muscles (*shoulder retractors*) pull, bracing the shoulders. There must be a balance in training between these to avoid the development of either a round-shouldered posture or a stiff 'military' bearing. The muscles which pull the arms downwards (*latissimus dorsi*) are important in lifting actions and although they are effectively worked with isolation movements, they should also be used in lifting actions to combine their action with the other lifting muscles such as the *gluteals* and *spinal extensors*. This type of functional action while working the muscles also rehearses the correct muscle sequencing for lifting and provides a more functional workout.

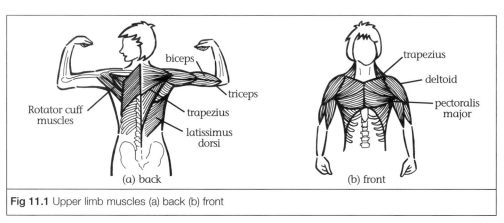

Fig 11.1 Upper limb muscles (a) back (b) front

The *deltoid* muscles form a 'cap' over the shoulder, attaching to the collar bone (clavicle) at the front and the shoulder blade (scapula) at the back. The deltoid has three parts, front, middle and back (anterior, lateral and posterior fibres) and all three must be worked. The deltoid is worked by lifting the arm away from the side of the body (abduction) and the front part is emphasised by lifting forwards (flexion-abduction), the side by lifting outwards (pure abduction) and the back by lifting backwards (extension-abduction) and pulling towards the body.

The shoulder is a ball and socket joint held together by powerful ligaments. These ligaments are assisted by the *rotator cuff* muscles which twist the arm inwards (medial rotation) and outwards (lateral rotation). The twisting action may be worked in isolation with a pulley or dumb-bell, or in combination with shoulder movements such as abduction in lateral raise movements for example.

The *biceps* muscle bends the arm and the *triceps* straightens the arm. Although they work on the arm, both muscles also affect the shoulder, the biceps pulling the arm forwards (shoulder flexion) and the triceps pulling it back (shoulder extension). Isolation movements such as arm curls and triceps extension actions will target the muscles, but combining elbow and shoulder movements such as dips and chinning actions will more effectively work the whole of the muscle.

The forearm muscles are also important, especially with the incidence of conditions such as tennis elbow and golfer's elbow (p. 204). The muscles will be worked in weight training simply through the gripping action used in training. However, again balance is important and if the *flexors* bending the wrist are stronger than the *extensors* straightening the wrist, the weaker group must be strengthened and the stronger tighter muscle stretched.

CHEST

BENCH PRESS (BARBELL)

Goal To strengthen the pectoral and triceps muscles.

Technique Position a barbell on the rack of a gym bench and check that the collars are tight and the barbell is in a central position on the rack. Your training partner should stand behind the barbell ready to pass the bar to you. Lie on a flat bench with your head resting on the bench surface. Your knees should be shoulder width apart and feet flat on the floor. Grip the bar (undergrasp) with your hands slightly wider than shoulder width apart. Lift the bar, assisted by your training partner, until the weight is positioned over the top of your chest at the level of your nipples. Inhale as you lower the weight onto your chest and exhale as you lift the bar again, locking your elbows out at the top position. Pause and then repeat the action.

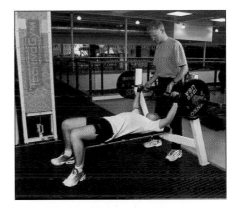

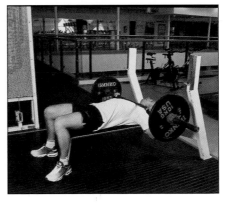

Points to note The bench press demands a fairly high degree of flexibility from the shoulder joints (anterior capsule)

and chest muscles (pectoralis major and anterior deltoid). If the stretch is uncomfortable do not lower the bar fully onto your chest, or use the machine chest press (p. 113) where the range of motion may be limited.

Some people find that placing the feet on the floor causes the back to arch so that the lumbar hollow (lordosis) is increased. If this is the case the feet may be drawn up and placed flat on the bench to flatten the lumbar spine. Although this greatly reduces the stress imposed on the lumbar region, it also reduces the general body stability. For this reason this technique must only be performed where your training partner is present as a 'spotter'.

Finally, as with all pressing actions, stress can build up on the back of the elbow (olecranon process). This usually occurs where the lift is performed rapidly and the elbow snapped back into hyperextension. To avoid this, the weight must be kept under control at all times, and the elbow straightened at the end of the movement, but not pressed backwards.

INCLINED BENCH PRESS

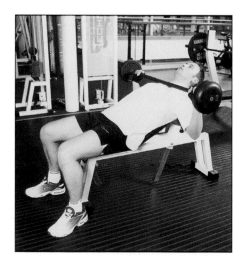

Goal To strengthen the pectoral and triceps muscles, placing emphasis on the upper part of the pectoral muscles (clavicular fibres).

Technique Position a barbell on the rack of a gym bench and check that the collars are tight and the barbell is in a central position on the rack. Your training partner should stand behind the barbell ready to pass the bar to you. Lie on an inclined bench with your head resting on the bench surface. Your knees should be shoulder width apart and feet flat on the floor. Grip the bar (under-grasp) with your hands slightly wider than shoulder width apart. Lift the bar, assisted by your training partner, until the weight is positioned over the top of your chest just above the level of your nipples. Inhale as you lower the weight onto your chest and exhale as you lift the bar again, locking your elbows out at the top position. Pause and then repeat the action.

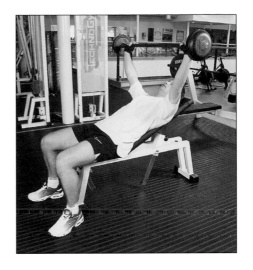

Points to note   In addition to those points noted for the general bench press above, the inclined bench press introduces a further challenge as the bar is moving at a diagonal. The combination of vertical and horizontal motion of the bar takes greater control and has a greater potential for injury through poor technique. For this reason, less weight is used with the inclined bench press than the general bench press, and adherence to good form is essential.

DECLINED BENCH PRESS

Goal To strengthen the pectoral and triceps muscles, placing emphasis on the lower part of the pectoral muscles (sternal fibres).

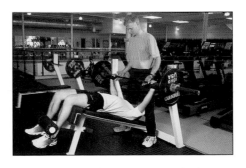

Technique   Position a barbell on the rack of a gym bench and check that the collars are tight and the barbell is in a central position on the rack. Your training partner should stand behind the barbell ready to pass the bar to you. Lie on a declined bench with your head resting on the bench surface. Your knees should be either shoulder width apart and feet flat on the floor, or on the bench with your feet hooked under the declined bench rollers. Grip the bar (undergrasp) with your hands slightly wider than shoulder width

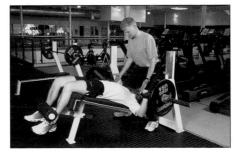

apart. Lift the bar, assisted by your training partner, until the weight is positioned over the top of your chest just below the level of your nipples. Inhale as you lower the weight onto your chest and exhale as you lift the bar again, locking your elbows out at the top position. Pause and then repeat the action.

Points to note As with the inclined bench press above, the declined press introduces a further challenge as the bar is moving at a diagonal. The combination of vertical and horizontal motion of the bar takes greater control and has a greater potential for injury through poor technique.

DUMB-BELL PRESS

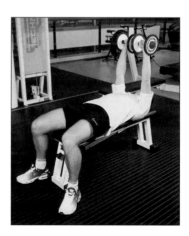

Goal To strengthen the pectoral muscles and triceps, and challenge coordination by using individual arm motion.

Technique Lie on a flat bench with your knees apart and feet flat on the floor. Have your training partner pass you two dumb-bells (one at a time) and hold them above your chest with your arms locked out straight. Inhale and slowly lower the dumb-bells, allowing your elbows to move outwards just below the level of your shoulders. Pause in the lower position and then press your arms out straight again as you exhale.

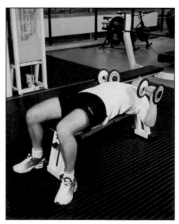

Points to note This action can place a significant stretch on the chest muscles and ribs. If you find this uncomfortable, limit the downwards motion by not allowing your elbows to sink down as far. If you find this difficult to control, have your training partner 'spot' you by placing one hand beneath each of the elbows as you perform the exercise.

SEATED CHEST PRESS

Goal To strengthen the chest muscles (pectorals) and the muscles on the back of the arm (triceps) from an easily accessible sitting position.

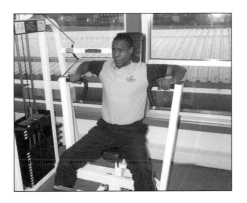

Technique Sit on the seat of the machine, adjusting it for comfort, and select an appropriate weight. Grip the machine handles, inhale and as you exhale press the handles forwards, straightening your arms. Pause and then lower the machine arms under control.

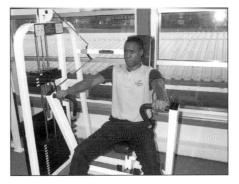

Points to note As you press the machine arms forwards be careful not to shrug or bunch your shoulders. Maintain the distance between your ear and shoulder throughout the movement. Many machines have an assistance pedal which when pressed with the foot will take some of the weight, making it easier to get into and out of the machine.

DUMB-BELL FLYE

Goal To strengthen and stretch the chest muscles (pectorals) while expanding the rib cage and increasing the volume of air taken into the lungs.

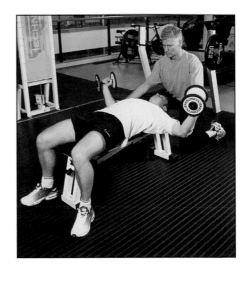

Technique Lie on a flat bench with your knees apart and feet flat on the floor. Have your training partner pass you two light dumb-bells (one at a time) and hold them above your chest with your arms unlocked and slightly bent. Slowly lower the dumb-bells and allow your elbows to move outwards and upwards towards your head in an arc.

As you do this, breathe in (inhale) and expand your rib cage. Pause in the fully stretched position and then return.

Points to note This action places an intense stretch on the chest muscles and ribs. If you find this uncomfortable, limit the downwards motion by not allowing your elbows to sink down as far. If this is difficult to control, have your training partner 'spot' you by placing one hand beneath each of the elbows as you perform the exercise.

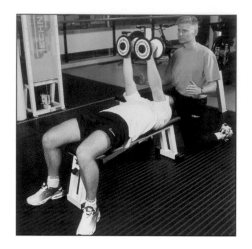

CABLE CROSSOVER (PECS)

Goal To strengthen the chest (pectoral) muscles and muscles beneath the arms (latissimus dorsi) from the standing position.

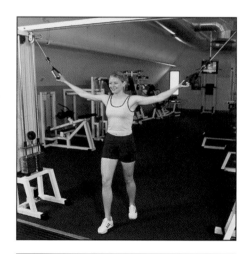

Technique Stand between two weight columns (high/low pulley) and grasp the 'D' handle of each unit in one hand, arms held out to the side. Take up a short lunge stance, with one foot slightly in front of the other to aid balance. Inhale and, as you exhale, bring your arms downwards and forwards (flexion-adduction) in front of your waist. Pause in this lower position and then release the weight under control.

Points to note The lowering (eccentric) component of this exercise is as important as the lifting component (concentric). Make sure that you lower the weight under control, avoiding any tendency to drop the weight or allow it to lower uncontrolled.

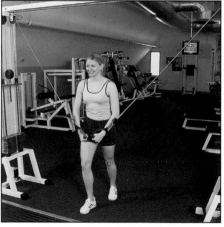

UPPER BACK

LAT PULL DOWN

Goal To exercise the muscles of the upper/side of the back (latissimus dorsi), with an emphasis on widening them.

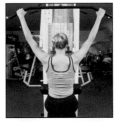
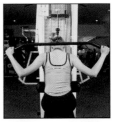
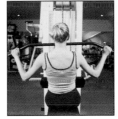
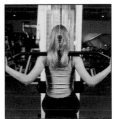

Technique Adjust the machine weight, stool height and roller height before beginning the exercise. Take a wide grip (overgrasp) on the bar and sit on the machine stool, hooking your knees beneath the rollers of the machine. As you exhale, pull the bar downwards and across the shoulders. Pause in the lower position and then allow the bar to raise again as the weight lowers under control.

Points to note Placing the bar behind the neck demands a reasonably high level of shoulder flexibility (lateral rotation). If you find this uncomfortable, take the bar in front of you to the top of your breastbone instead. Make sure you tie your hair back if you pull the bar behind your neck. It will trap on the moving cable and cause injury (see bottom right).

CLOSE GRIP PULL DOWN

Goal To exercise the muscles of the upper/side of the back (latissimus dorsi), with an emphasis on thickening them.

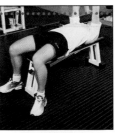
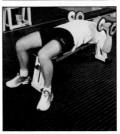

Technique Adjust the machine weight, stool height and roller height before beginning the exercise. Take a narrow grip (undergrasp) on the bar and sit on the machine stool, hooking your knees beneath the rollers of the machine. Pull the bar downwards to the top of your breastbone in a 'chinning' action. Pause in the lower position and then allow the bar to raise again, as the weight lowers under control.

Points to note   As you pull the bar downwards it will pass close to your face. Make sure that you pay close attention to its movement to avoid the possibility of injury.

SINGLE ARM DUMB-BELL ROW

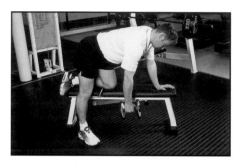

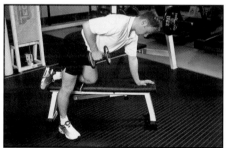

Goal   To exercise the muscles under the arm (latisimus dorsi) and those on the back of the arm and shoulder (posterior deltoid and triceps).

Technique   Half kneel on a gym bench with your left knee and left hand on the bench, right foot on the floor. Grip a dumb-bell in your right hand and, as you exhale, pull the dumb-bell towards your chest and side of the body. Pause in this upper position and then lower once more.

Points to note   Make sure that you maintain your back alignment throughout this movement. Avoid the temptation to twist your trunk or sway from the waist. As you pull the dumb-bell towards you, imagine that you are trying to brush the side of your chest with it.

UPRIGHT BARBELL ROW

Goal   To exercise the shoulder shrugging and lifting muscles (deltoid and upper trapezius).

Technique   Grip a barbell with your hands 10–15 cm apart and overgrasp. Stand with your feet comfortably astride, the barbell resting on your waist or upper thighs. As you exhale, lift the barbell in an upward motion, keeping it close to your body. Lead the move-

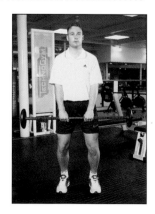

ment with your elbows and keep your elbows above your wrists throughout the movement. Stop when the bar reaches the upper part of your breastbone (sternum) and then lower the weight under control and repeat.

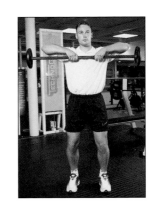

Points to note As you lift the weight, leading with your wrist, the amount of movement (flexion) required from the wrist increases as the bar goes up. If you find this painful, stop the bar at the lower part of your breastbone rather than the upper part. If you use a lighter weight and higher reps (circuit weight training), change the breathing around. Inhale as you lift to expand your upper rib cage and exhale as you lower the bar, allowing your rib cage to sink back.

SINGLE ARM PULLEY ROW

Goal To exercise the muscles under the arm (latisimus dorsi) and those on the back of the arm and shoulder (posterior deltoid and triceps) from a standing position.

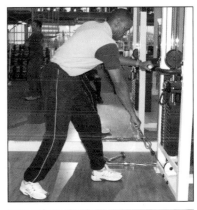

Technique Stand in a lunge position with your left leg forwards. Grip the handle of the machine with your right hand and place your left hand on your left knee for support. Exhale and raise the weight by pulling your right hand towards your body in a rowing action, aiming to scrape the side of your body with your hand. As you pull the machine handle in towards yourself, slightly brace your right shoulder and pause in this tightened position. Lower the weight under control and then repeat with the left arm, this time placing the right leg forwards.

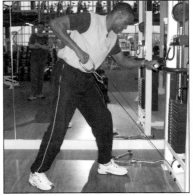

Points to note The action is usually restricted to your arm and shoulder only, with the trunk immobile. However, to work the trunk rotators (oblique abdominals) at the same time, twist the trunk to the right as you pull the right arm towards you. Return to the forward-facing position as the weight is lowered.

SEATED ROW (LOW PULLEY)

Goal To strengthen the shoulder bracing muscles (retractors) and those under the arm (latissimus dorsi) while maintaining optimal spinal alignment in sitting.

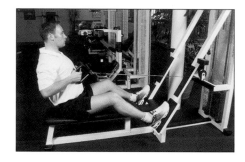

Technique Sit on the floor in front of the low pulley unit, knees bent and feet flat on the floor. Grip the handles of the machine in each hand and, as you exhale, pull them towards you in a rowing action, bracing the shoulder slightly and straightening the shoulders as you do so. Pause in the inward position and then lower the weight under control, maintaining spinal alignment.

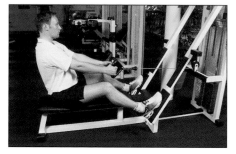

Points to note If too large a weight is used, the spine may be pulled forwards into flexion and can remain in this position throughout the movement. The action then simply hinges on the hip, with the arms providing secondary power. To avoid this, use lower weights and focus closely on optimal technique.

SEATED ROW (MACHINE)

Goal To strengthen the shoulder-bracing muscles (retractors) and those under the arm (latissimus dorsi) with the chest and spine supported throughout the movement.

Technique Adjust the seat height and chest pad of the machine for comfort. Sit on the machine and reach forwards for the machine handles. Straighten and lengthen your spine by sitting tall, and then pull the machine handles towards you in a rowing action as you exhale. Slightly brace your shoulders at the innermost point of the movement and then lower the weight under control.

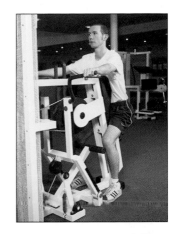

Points to note If the chest pad is too far from the machine, the spine will bend as you overreach with your arms. To avoid this, adjust the chest pad so that your arms are very slightly bent at the start of the movement.

If you use a lighter weight and higher reps (circuit weight training) you can reverse the breathing, breathing in as you pull the machine handles towards you to expand your chest and breathing out as you lower the weight allowing your chest to relax.

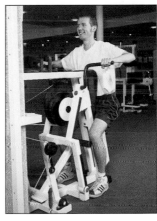

PULL OVER

Goal To work the latissimus dorsi muscle beneath the arm and expand the rib cage at the same time.

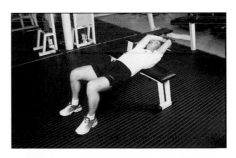

Technique Lie across a gym bench with your shoulder blades on the bench, feet flat on the floor and astride. Ask your training partner to pass you a dumb-bell and grasp it in both hands. Keep your arms slightly bent (elbows unlocked or 'soft') and inhale as you reach up and overhead with your whole arm moving as a single unit. Pause in the position of maximum comfortable stretch and then bring the arms back into the starting position, exhaling as you do so. Choose a

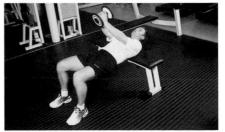

stable bench when performing this exercise to ensure it does not tip over. If the bench rocks, turn it around and lie along it rather than across it.

Points to note This exercise expands the rib cage and stretches the shoulders quite significantly. If you find this uncomfortable, ask your training partner to 'spot' the weight by kneeling behind you and supporting the dumb-bell as it moves into its lowest position.

MACHINE PULL OVER

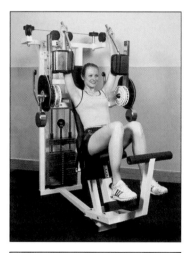

Goal To work the latissimus dorsi muscles beneath the arm in a supported sitting position.

Technique Adjust the seat of the machine so that the pivot point of the machine arm is level with your shoulder, and fasten the machine seatbelt around your waist. Use the assistance pedal to take the weight of the machine and hold the machine bar with your forearms on the padded supports. Inhale and reach above your head and backwards expanding your chest as you do so. Exhale and draw the bar downwards towards your waist. Control the weight throughout the action, and do not allow the machine arm to swing.

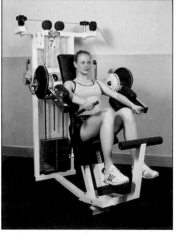

Points to note Most machine pull over units place a significant stretch on the chest, thoracic spine and latissimus muscles. If this stretch is too much for you, use the assistance pedal to take the weight at the end of the movement, and perform the action within your mid range only.

BODYTONING

SHOULDER RETRACTION MACHINE

Goal To strengthen and shorten the muscles between the shoulder blades (retractors).

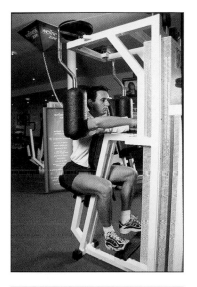

Technique Sit on the machine and adjust the seat height so that your spine is straight and shoulders aligned (not bunched up or elevated) when you are holding the machine bars. Using a light weight, inhale and draw the bars backwards, squeezing your shoulder blades together as you do so. Pause in the fully contracted position and then lower the weight once more.

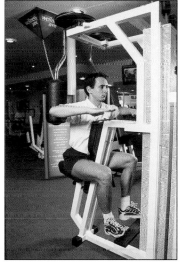

Points to note In a round-shouldered posture (p. 44) the shoulder retractor muscles are often lax, allowing the shoulder blades to move apart excessively. To correct this, these muscles have to be shortened as well as strengthened. Muscles can be shortened by working them in their inner range, and holding the position. In the case of the shoulder retractors, the shortened position is with the shoulder blades drawn together (braced). To achieve postural correction with this exercise when the weight has been lifted, hold the inner position for 10–15 seconds using a light weight.

SHOULDERS

SHOULDER SHRUG WITH BARBELL

Goal To work the upper trapezius muscle between the shoulders and neck, with secondary work to the shoulder bracing muscles (retractors).

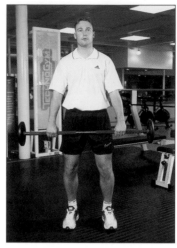

Technique Grip a barbell overgrasp, with your arms slightly wider than shoulder width apart. Allow the weight to draw your shoulders downwards (shoulder depression), increasing the distance between your ears and shoulders. Keeping your arms straight (elbows locked), shrug your shoulders to lift them up towards your ears. Hold this tight position and then lower. Breathe normally throughout the movement.

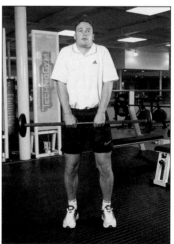

Points to note Although this is a strengthening exercise it can also be used to allow the upper trapezius muscle to relax. Where the muscle is tight and thickened, use a very light weight (just the bar alone may be sufficient depending on your body build). Lift the weight in a shrugging action for a count of two and then lower the weight to a count of four, allowing the weight to pull your shoulders right down and stretch the upper trapezius muscles.

SHOULDER SHRUG WITH DUMB-BELL

Goal To work the upper trapezius muscle between the shoulders and neck, and the shoulder bracing muscles (retractors).

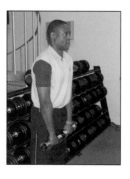

Technique Grip two dumb-bells overgrasp with your arms slightly wider than shoulder width apart. Allow the weights to draw your shoulders downwards and forwards (shoulder depression and protraction), increasing the distance between your ears and shoulders, and allowing your shoulder blades to move apart. Keeping your arms straight (elbows locked), exhale and shrug your shoulders to lift them up towards your ears, and brace them at the same time, squeezing the shoulder blades together. Hold this tight position and then lower. Breathe normally throughout the movement.

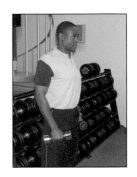

Points to note The action of combined shoulder shrugging and shoulder bracing gives the movement a circular appearance, rolling the shoulder up and back in a semicircle.

SHOULDER PRESS WITH BARBELL (BEHIND NECK)

Goal To strengthen the deltoid muscles of the shoulder and the triceps on the back of the arm.

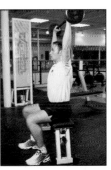
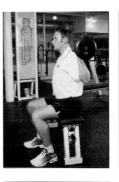

Technique Sit astride a gym bench with your back aligned (sit 'tall'), or use the back rest of a bench. Ask your training partner to pass you a barbell and rest it across your shoulders. Grip the bar undergrasp using a comfortable width grip. Inhale and, as you exhale, look down slightly to nod your head and press the bar upwards straightening your arms. Lower the weight under control.

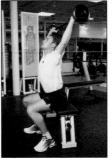
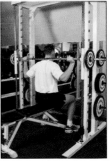

Points to note As you lift the weight, there is a tendency to angle the body forwards and push the arms backwards to gain extra purchase from the muscles (see bottom left). If this occurs, the weight is too heavy. Reduce the weight and keep the body aligned throughout the action. Ensure that the bar travels in a vertical path rather than obliquely. Use a lifting rack to enable you to control the barbell more accurately (see bottom right).

SHOULDER PRESS WITH BARBELL (IN FRONT OF HEAD)

Goal To strengthen the deltoid muscles of the shoulder and the triceps on the back of the arm.

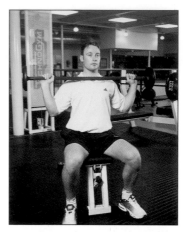

Technique Sit astride a gym bench with your back aligned (sit 'tall'), or use the back rest of the bench. Ask your training partner to pass you a barbell and rest it on your upper chest and shoulders. Grip the bar undergrasp, using a comfortable width grip. Inhale and, as you exhale, press the bar directly upwards, straightening your arms. Lower the weight under control.

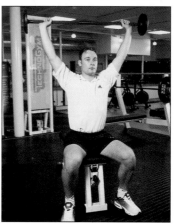

Points to note As you lift the weight, there is a tendency to overhollow the back and push the bar more from the chest, gaining extra power from the large chest muscles (pectorals). If this occurs, the weight is too heavy. Reduce the weight and keep the body aligned throughout the action. Ensure that the bar travels in a vertical path rather than obliquely. This exercise can also be performed standing (p. 186).

SHOULDER PRESS WITH DUMB-BELL

Goal To strengthen the deltoid muscles of the shoulder and the triceps at the back of the arm, while introducing single arm coordination

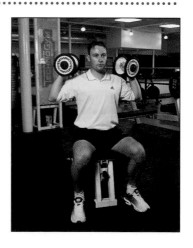

Technique Sit astride a gym bench with your back aligned ('sit tall'). Ask your training partner to pass the two dumb-bells, one at a time, and hold them on your shoulders. As you exhale press the dumb-bells overhead slightly turning your forearms to keep your knuckles facing outwards. Pause in the overhead position and then lower.

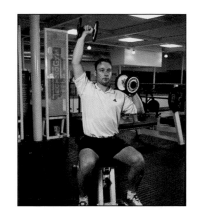

Points to note This exercise may either be performed with one arm at a time (alternative dumb-bell shoulder press) or with both arms together. When the arms are straightened, aim for the upper arm to lie over the ear, indicating that the arm is verticle. If your shoulders and thoracic spine are very tight, your arm may lie in front of your ear showing that you need to practice some stretching exercises for this area (Fig 8.4. p .76).

MACHINE SHOULDER PRESS

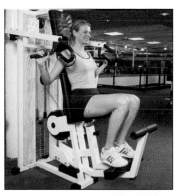

Goal To strengthen the major shoulder muscles (deltoids) and the muscles on the back of the arms (triceps).

Technique Sit on the machine seat and adjust the seat height so that the bar rests approximately one hand breadth above the shoulder. Grip the bar and exhale as you press the bar overhead. Straighten the arms, but do not lock them rapidly (elbow *hyperextension*) and then lower the bar under control.

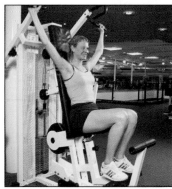

Points to note Most press machines offer a number of alternative handles for different hand positions. A wider grip throws greater stress on the deltoids and less on the triceps as the arms are travelling more obliquely as the bar moves. A narrower grip emphasises the triceps as the bar is travelling more vertically.

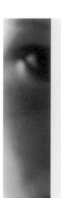

Elbow strain

All pressing actions can place excessive stress on the elbows if they are performed rapidly. This is because rapid actions allow the elbow to lock out too far (hyperextend) and squeeze the bone on the back of the elbow (olecranon). The result can be a painful swollen elbow, with the pain focused on the back of the joint. If this occurs, rest completely and see a qualified physiotherapist. When you resume training, use light weights and pay close attention to your technique.

MACHINE LATERAL RAISE

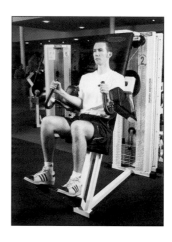

Goal To strengthen the deltoid muscles of the shoulder, emphasising the outer portion (lateral fibres).

Technique Sit on the machine seat and adjust the seat height so that the pivot points of the machine arms are aligned with the centre of your shoulders. Grip the machine handles and as you exhale, raise your arms, leading with your elbows until your arms are horizontal. Pause in this upper position and then lower.

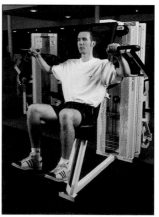

Points to note This is an isolation movement which also restricts the normal twisting (rotation) action of the shoulder joint. If you are prone to shoulder problems (clicking and catching pain) it may hurt. If it does, use the lateral raise with pulley (p. 127) instead, as this allows the ball and socket joint of the shoulder to rotate freely.

BODYTONING

LATERAL RAISE WITH DUMB-BELL

Goal To work the deltoid (shoulder) muscles in isolation.

Technique Hold a light dumb-bell in each hand. Stand with your feet shoulder width apart and knees slightly bent (soft). Keeping your elbows straight but not completely locked out, inhale and take your arms out to the side and above your head (shoulder abduction). As you do this, allow your arms to turn naturally, so that the thumbs face the ceiling. Pause in the upward position and then lower under control.

Points to note If you are using heavier weights and focusing on deltoid bulk, you can limit the movement, taking your arms to the horizontal position only. In this case you should lead the movement with your knuckles (shoulder medial rotation) rather than your thumbs (shoulder lateral rotation).

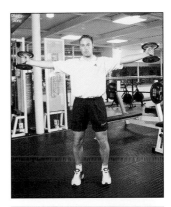

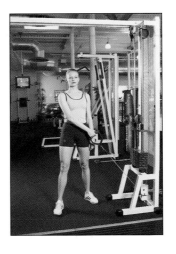

LATERAL RAISE WITH PULLEY

Goal To work the deltoid (shoulder) muscles and rotator cuff (shoulder twisting) muscles.

Technique Hold the handle of a low pulley machine in your right hand. Stand one foot forward in a lunge position, and place your left hand on the frame of the pulley machine (be careful not to place your hand near the moving weight). Keeping your elbows straight but not completely locked out, inhale and take your arm out to the side, turning your whole arm so that your thumb faces the ceiling. Pause in the upward position and then lower under control as you exhale.

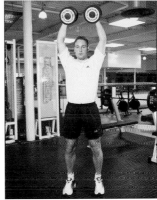

Points to note Try to isolate the movement to the shoulder alone, do not allow the trunk to twist or bend.

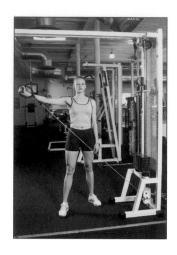

PULLEY SHOULDER ROTATION (OUTWARDS)

Goal To work the rotator cuff (shoulder twisting) muscles in isolation.

Technique Stand or kneel side on to an adjustable pulley machine and grip the pulley handle with your right hand. Your left hand can rest on the machine frame for balance. Bend the elbow of your right arm and tuck it into the side of your body just above the hip. Keep the elbow bent to 90° throughout the movement, and twist the whole arm outwards (lateral rotation) so that your forearm moves horizontally. Pause in the outermost position and then lower the weight. Breathe normally throughout the movement.

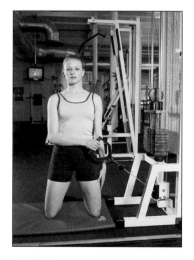

Points to note You will need to adjust your foot and body position at the beginning of the exercise to take up the slack in the machine cable and make sure the weight resistance is acting throughout the whole movement.

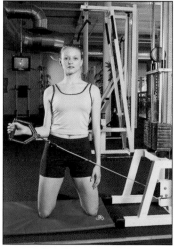

PULLEY SHOULDER ROTATION (INWARDS)

Goal To work the rotator cuff (shoulder twisting) muscles in isolation.

Technique Stand or kneel side on to an adjustable pulley machine and grip the pulley handle with your right hand, your left hand can rest on the machine frame for balance. Bend the elbow of your right arm and tuck into the side of your body just above the hip. Keep the elbow bent to 90° throughout the movement, and twist the whole arm inwards (medial rotation) so that your forearm moves horizontally. Pause in the innermost position and then lower the weight. Breathe normally throughout the movement.

Points to note You will need to adjust your foot and body position at the beginning of the exercise to take up the slack in the machine cable and make sure the weight resistance is acting throughout the whole movement.

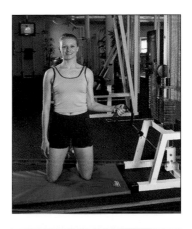

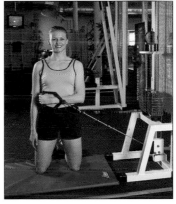

DUMB-BELL SHOULDER ROTATION

Goal To work the rotator cuff (shoulder twisting) muscles in isolation.

Technique Lie on your right side on a gym mat and grip a light dumb-bell in your left hand. Bend your left elbow and tuck into the side of your body just above the hip. Keep the elbow bent to 90° throughout the movement, and twist the whole left arm outwards (lateral rotation) so that your forearm moves towards the vertical. Pause in the outermost position and then lower the weight. Breathe normally throughout the movement.

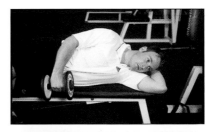

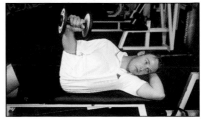

Points to note Initially the amount of movement upwards may be quite small. Part of the function of this exercise, however, is to increase the range of motion available to the shoulder, so the upwards movement that you can achieve should increase over time.

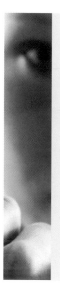

Rotator cuff muscles

The rotator cuff muscles twist the shoulder inwards (medial rotation) and outwards (lateral rotation). They are important muscles deep under the skin surface which in addition to their twisting action actually help to keep the ball of the shoulder joint securely in the socket. After a shoulder dislocation injury, for example, the rotator cuff muscles may be very weak, requiring restrengthening under the supervision of the physiotherapist. The rotator cuff also works to guide the bones within the shoulder joint as they move. Poor tone in the rotator cuff muscles can therefore give rise to injury, causing trapping or pinching (*impingement*) of shoulder structures. The inclusion of some rotator cuff work in a gym programme is therefore useful for general shoulder health.

FRONT RAISE WITH DUMB-BELL

Goal To work the front portion of the deltoid (shoulder) muscles in isolation.

Technique Hold a dumb-bell in each hand and stand with the knees slightly unlocked (soft) and spine aligned. Keeping the elbow slightly bent but arm stiff, lift one arm upwards leading with the knuckles. With a light weight (for muscle tone) the arm raises overhead, and with a heavier weight (for muscle bulk) the arm stops at the horizontal position and then lowers. Repeat the movement with the other arm, raising one dumb-bell as the other lowers. Breathe normally throughout the movement.

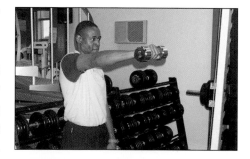

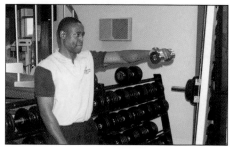

Points to note If you find yourself arching your back and leaning backwards, you have chosen a weight which is too heavy. Reduce the weight and use one dumb-bell only, gripping the frame of a gym machine with the other hand for balance.

ARMS

ARM CURL WITH LOW PULLEY

Goal To exercise the arm-bending muscles (biceps and brachialis).

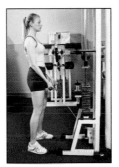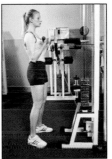

Technique Grip the straight bar of a low pulley machine with both hands and stand facing the machine with your back straight and knees slightly bent. Exhale and bend your arms, keeping your elbows tucked into the sides of your body. Pause in the upper position and then lower the weight under control.

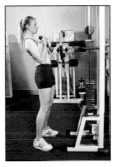

Points to note The elbow does not bend and straighten in a straight line, but at a slight angle, making a straight bar feel slightly awkward with heavier weights. Where this occurs use a Z shaped bar called an EZ ('easy') bar, where the grip is angled slightly. Make sure you do not lean backwards as you lift the weights as this can stress the lower back (see bottom photo).

ARM CURL WITH BARBELL

Goal To exercise the arm-bending muscles (biceps and brachialis) using a free weight.

Technique Grip a barbell with both hands and stand with your back straight and knees slightly bent. Exhale and bend your arms keeping your elbows tucked into the sides of your body. Pause in the upper position and then lower the weight under control.

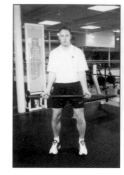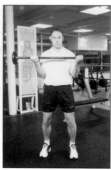

Points to note Try to avoid body sway as you perform this exercise as it reduces the work of the arm muscles, throwing it instead onto the trunk. As you use heavier weights, reduce body sway by taking up a lunge position with one foot in front of the other. As the weight moves in your arms, transfer your weight onto and off the front leg rather than bending your back.

ARM CURL WITH DUMB-BELL

Goal To exercise the arm-bending muscles (biceps and brachialis) using single arms.

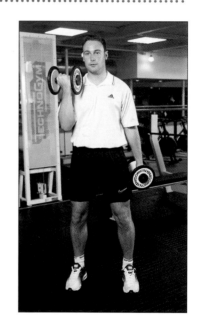

Technique Grip a dumb-bell in each hand and stand with your back straight and knees slightly bent. Exhale and bend one arm, keeping your elbow tucked into the side of your body. Pause in the upper position and then lower the weight under control. Repeat the movement with the other arm, raising one arm as the other lowers.

Points to note As the arm raises, allow the forearm to twist slightly, taking the weight from a knuckles sideways to a knuckles downwards position. This action (forearm supination) is a secondary action of the biceps and will help to give the biceps a full workout.

PREACHER CURL MACHINE

Goal To intensify the work on the arm flexor muscles (biceps and brachialis).

Technique Sit on the stool of the

preacher curl unit and adjust the pad so that the pivot point of the machine bar is level with your elbow joint. Grip the bar in a comfortable position and bend the arm, pulling the bar upwards and inwards towards your shoulders. Squeeze the final few degrees of movement out at the end of the range (peak contraction – see p. 95), pause and then lower the weight under control. Breathe normally throughout the movement.

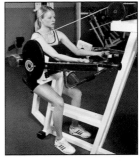

Points to note   The biceps muscle of the arm has an action over both the shoulder (flexion) and the elbow (flexion and supination). The preacher curl exercise, although intense, only works the muscle with elbow movement. For a complete long-term workout, therefore, other biceps exercises involving shoulder motion must be included.

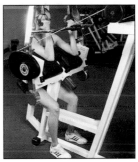

PREACHER CURL WITH BARBELL

Goal   To intensify the work on the arm flexor muscles (biceps and brachialis) using a free weight.

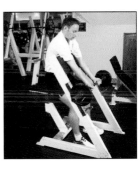

Technique   Sit on the stool of the preacher curl unit and adjust the pad so that the arm is fully supported but able to move unhindered. Grip the barbell in a comfortable position and bend the arm pulling the bar upwards and inwards towards your shoulders. Squeeze the final few degrees of movement out at the end of the range, pause and then lower the weight under control. Breathe normally throughout the movement.

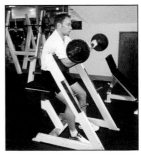

Points to note   The arm does not move in a straight line as it bends, but through a

UPPER LIMB WEIGHT TRAINING EXERCISES

slight arc. For this reason a straight bar becomes uncomfortable when heavier weights are used and an angled bar (EZ bar) should be used instead.

ISOLATION CURL WITH DUMB-BELL

Goal To work the arm flexor muscles (biceps and brachialis) using a single arm action.

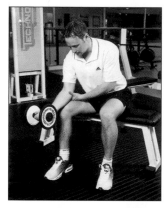

Technique Sit on a gym bench holding a dumb-bell in your right hand. Place your right elbow against your right thigh for support, and bend your arm pulling the dumb-bell upwards and inwards towards your left shoulder. Squeeze the final few degrees of movement out at the end of the range, pause and then lower the weight under control. Breath normally throughout the movement.

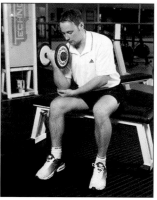

Points to note The action of the biceps is arm bending (flexion) combined with forearm twisting (supination). With this exercise, a more complete workout on the biceps is therefore achieved by twisting the forearm from a position of knuckles to the side to knuckles facing down as the arm is bent.

CLOSE GRIP PULL-UP

Goal To work the arm flexors and shoulder extensors simultaneously against body weight.

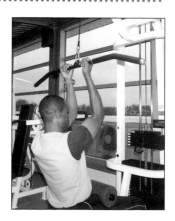

Technique Grip a chinning bar undergrasp, with the hands shoulder width apart. Exhale and pull the body upwards using arm power alone until the chin passes over the bar. Lower the body again under control and inhale.

BODYTONING

11

Points to note This is an extremely intense movement, and users often swing the body to gain momentum and make the exercise easier. However, if the exercise is too difficult a safer alternative is to ask your training partner to spot you (p. 7). You should cross your legs at the calves while your training partner stands behind you. As you pull up your partner lifts your body slightly, gripping your shins. At the top position they release their grip and allow you to control your body weight as you descend.

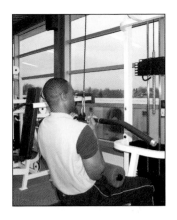

CHINNING MOVEMENT - MACHINE ASSISTED

Goal To perform an assisted chinning action without a training partner.

Technique Adjust the machine weight for the amount of assistance you require. If a larger weight is chosen, more assistance is provided, making the exercise easier. Place your knees or feet on the step of the machine and grip the chinning bar undergrasp with the hands shoulder width apart. Exhale and pull your body upwards using arm power alone until the chin passes over the bar. Lower the body again under control as you inhale.

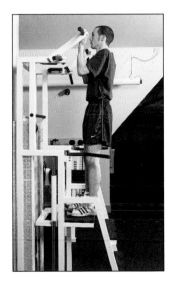

Points to note Chinning movements are often thought to be for advanced users only. However, the chinning action combines both elbow and shoulder movements, and works a large number of muscles. For this reason it is an important movement to include. In weaker subjects the exercise is still very useful and should be used even though large poundages may be required to counterbalance your body weight for assistance.

OVERHEAD TRICEPS EXTENSION WITH DUMB-BELL

Goal To work the triceps muscles in isolation from a fully stretched position.

Technique Sit astride a gym bench. Hold a dumb-bell in both hands, the web of the finger/thumb of each hand at the dumb-bell handle and the hands flat against the dumb-bell plate. Take the dumb-bell behind the head to lightly touch the centre of the shoulders. Your elbows should be held in to brush the sides of your head. Straighten the arms to reach the dumb-bell overhead, pause and then lower the weight under control. Breathe normally throughout the movement.

Points to note With a heavy weight the position of the dumb-bell overhead introduces a potential risk. For this reason always use your training partner to spot the movement if you are uncomfortable lifting the weight you have chosen with one hand.

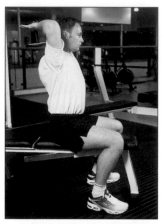

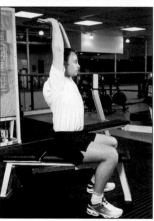

OVERHEAD TRICEPS EXTENSION WITH DUMB-BELL (SINGLE-HANDED)

Goal To work the triceps muscles in isolation, using a single-handed technique.

Technique Sit astride a gym bench. Hold a dumb-bell in your right hand and take the dumb-bell behind your head to lightly touch the centre of the shoulders. Reach up with your left hand and rest the elbow of the right arm in your left palm to steady the arm. Your right elbow should be held in to brush the right side of your head. Straighten your right

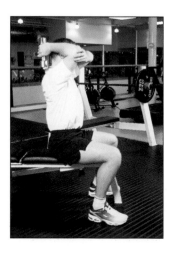

arm to reach the dumb-bell overhead, pause and then lower the weight under control. Repeat the movement with your left arm. Breathe normally throughout the movement.

Points to note As you stop the shoulder from contributing to the movement, the weight lifted is far lighter than can be used in non-supported movements.

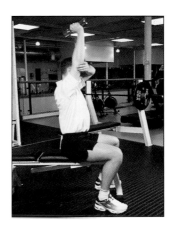

TRICEPS PUSH DOWN FROM A HIGH PULLEY

Goal To strengthen the triceps in isolation from a neutral shoulder position.

Technique Stand facing a high pulley machine with your knees slightly bent and back aligned. Grip the bar (overgrasp) and tuck your elbows into your sides. Press downwards to straighten your arms, pausing at the end position and then allow your arms to bend again under control. Breathe normally throughout the movement.

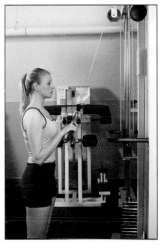

Points to note Several bars are available for this exercise. A straight bar is fine for lighter weights, but for heavier weights an angled bar is more comfortable as it twists (partially supinates) the forearm and allows the elbow to move more naturally. A knotted rope is also useful. Again it permits a more natural movement at the elbow, and has the additional advantage that it allows the hands to pass to the side of the body at the end of the movement. This creates shoulder extension (a secondary action of the triceps) and allows greater tension to be built up in the muscle.

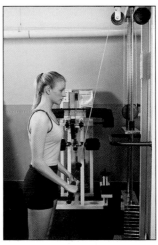

TRICEPS EXTENSION WITH A BARBELL

Goal To work the triceps in isolation from a fully stretched position using a free weight.

Technique Sit on a gym bench. Grip a barbell undergrasp with your hands one hand width apart. Take the bar overhead and hold your elbows into the side of your head. Allow your elbows to bend, taking the weight behind your head, and then straighten your arms again. Breathe normally throughout the movement.

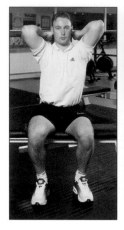
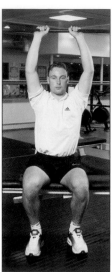

Points to note This exercise places a significant stress on the structures at the back of the elbow, most noticeably the tendon of the triceps muscle and the cushion (bursa) beneath it. If you get elbow pain with this movement, change to another triceps isolation exercise, such as the triceps kickback or triceps push down using a pulley.

TRICEPS EXTENSION WITH A LOW PULLEY

Goal To work the triceps in isolation from a fully stretched position using a pulley.

Technique Sit or kneel with your back towards a low pulley machine and ask your training partner to pass you the bar from the machine. Grip the bar undergrasp over your head with your hands one hand width apart. Hold your elbows into the side of your head. Allow your elbows to bend, taking the weight behind your head, and then straighten your arms again, exhaling as you do so.

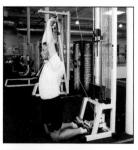
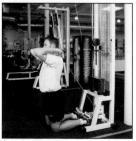

Points to note The starting position for this exercise is quite awkward due to the pull of the pulley machine. It is essential to have assistance lifting the bar overhead to avoid the possibility of the machine cable springing back into the machine.

TRICEPS EXTENSION MACHINE

Goal To strengthen the triceps with an isolation movement using a supported upper arm.

Technique Sit on the machine stool and place your upper arm on the machine pad, adjusting it for your body size. Grip the handles and press them forwards extending (straightening) your elbows as you do so. Pause in the straight position and then lower under control. Breathe normally throughout the movement, do not hold your breath.

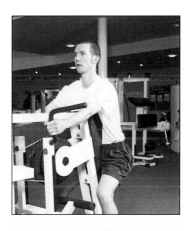

Points to note This action straightens the arm but does not allow twisting actions. If you find this uncomfortable, use an alternative exercise for the triceps such as triceps kickback (p.141) or triceps pushdown (p. 137).

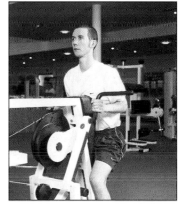

DIPS - FROM FRAME

Goal To work the triceps against full body weight resistance.

Technique Grip the handles of a dipping frame and use one leg to lift you into position. Inhale and lower yourself until your elbows are bent to 90°. Exhale and push yourself back to the starting position straightening your arms.

Points to note This movement places a significant stretch on the chest muscles (pectorals) and ribs. If you find this position uncomfortable limit your movement by placing one foot on the ground in the lower position.

DIPS - MACHINE ASSISTED

Goal To work the triceps against partial body weight resistance.

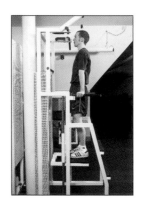

Technique Adjust the machine weight to provide a counterbalance to your own body weight. Grip the handles of a dipping machine and use the step support to lift you into position. Inhale and lower yourself until your elbows are bent to 90°. Exhale and push yourself back to the starting position, straightening your arms.

Points to note This movement places a significant stretch on the chest muscles (pectorals) and ribs. If you find this position uncomfortable limit your movement by placing one foot on the ground in the lower position. As this exercise works on a counterweight principle, selecting a larger weight will make the exercise easier.

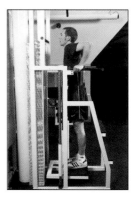

CLOSE GRIP BENCH DIP

Goal To work the triceps muscle at the back of the arm over the elbow and shoulder simultaneously.

Technique Stand with your back towards the narrow end of a gym bench (secured against the wall to avoid it slipping). Place your hands flat on the end of the bench with your fingers facing forwards, and your feet either on the floor or on another gym bench. Inhale and slowly lower yourself downwards, bending your arms until your elbows are at a 90° angle. Pause in this position and then push with your arms to bring yourself back to the starting position, exhaling as you do so.

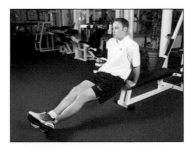

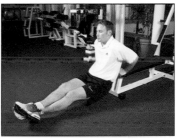

Points to note   This exercise places a significant compression and backward bending (extension) force on the wrist. If you find this uncomfortable, turn your hand so that your fingers point outwards, to reduce the demand for extension of the wrist.

TRICEPS KICKBACK

Goal   To work the triceps muscles in isolation single-handedly.

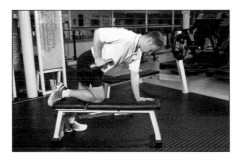

Technique   Grip a dumb-bell in your right hand and kneel on a gym bench with your right knee and left hand on the bench and left foot on the ground. Tuck your right elbow into your side and begin with your elbow bent to 90°. Keeping your elbow tucked in, straighten (extend) your arm, hold the straight position and then lower under control. Breathe normally throughout the movement.

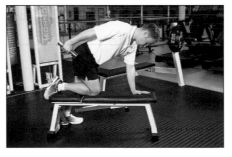

Points to note   The intensity of this exercise can be increased by lifting the straight arm slightly at the end of the movement (shoulder extension). This is because a secondary function of the triceps muscle is to extend the shoulder.

FOREARMS
WRIST CURL

Goal To strengthen the forearm bending (flexion) muscles in isolation.

Technique Sit on a gym bench holding a barbell (undergrasp) with your hands one hand width apart. Support your forearms on your knees. Roll the barbell downwards, straightening your fingers and pressing your wrists back (extension) until the bar reaches your finger tips. Roll the bar up your fingers again and bend (flex) your wrists. Breathe normally throughout the movement.

Points to note This action must be slow and controlled to avoid the chance of the barbell rolling out of the hand completely.

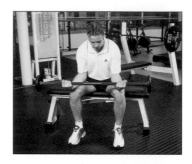
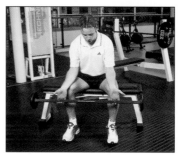

WRIST EXTENSION

Goal To strengthen the wrist straightening muscles (extensors) in isolation.

Technique Sit on a gym bench holding a barbell (overgrasp) with your hands one hand width apart. Support your elbows/fore-arms on your thighs. Lift your wrist up (extension) gripping the barbell and then allow the wrist to bend once more, angling down fully to a 90° bend at the wrist. Breathe normally throughout the movement.

Points to note Lifting your forearms off your thighs at the point of maximum wrist extension will intensify the movement by working the upper forearm muscle (brachio-radialis) which crosses the elbow.

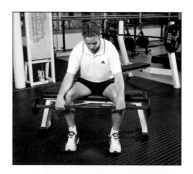
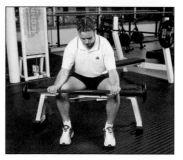

REVERSE CURL WITH BARB-BELL

Goal To work the wrist extensor muscles with the side upper forearm muscle (brachio-radialis).

Technique Grip a barbell (overgrasp) with your hands just wider than shoulder width apart. Tuck your elbows lightly into your sides. Bend your elbows and straighten them, keeping your knuckles facing upwards. Breathe normally throughout the movement.

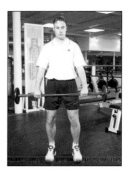

Points to note If you find one hand is noticeably stronger than the other, perform the same action using a dumb-bell in each hand.

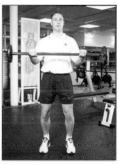

PRONATION/SUPINATION (HAMMER CURL)

Goal To work the arm twisting muscles (pronators and supinators).

Technique Remove the weight at one end of a dumb-bell and grip the bar in the right hand. Bend your right elbow to 90° and tuck your right arm into your side. Twist your forearm (keeping the rest of your arm still) so that the modified dumb-bell describes a vertical circle. Breathe normally throughout the movement.

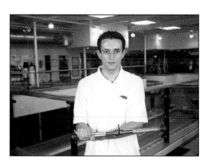

Points to note Instead of using a modified dumb-bell, a stick (brush handle) or unloaded bar may be used. Grip the bar at the end, and the leverage effect provides the overload.

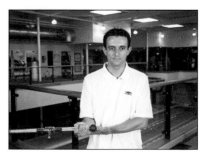

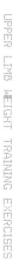

UPPER LIMB WEIGHT TRAINING EXERCISES

In addition to providing the impetus for locomotion (walking, running and jumping), the leg muscles also provide the power for lifting (Fig. 12.1). It is important therefore for a truly complete workout that some of the structured lifting techniques covered in chapter 17 are used. This is especially the case if you use lifting as part of your job, or if you are recovering from a back injury. Rehearsing good lifting techniques makes back injury less likely, and works the leg muscles together with those of the trunk in a more functional fashion.

The gluteal muscles are among the largest and most powerful muscles in the body. The *gluteus maximus* is the 'bum' muscle and works to pull the thigh bone backwards (extension of the femur). The muscle also works when the trunk is hinged forwards at

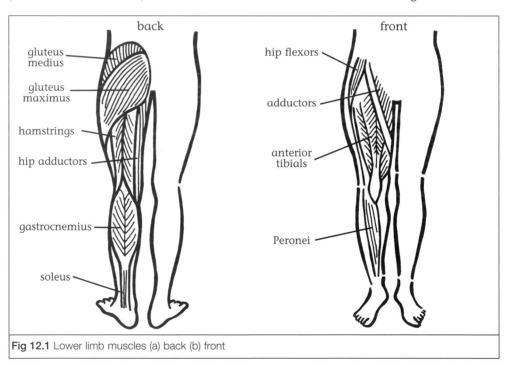

Fig 12.1 Lower limb muscles (a) back (b) front

the waist, as with a hip hinge action (p. 158). Both movements are important if the whole of the gluteus is to be targeted. The *gluteus medius* is a smaller muscle at the side of the hip. It acts to support your body weight when you stand on one leg, and so is targeted more effectively with single leg actions such as lunges.

The gluteal muscles are helped in their action of hip extension by the *hamstring* muscles which travel from the sitting bone down the back of the leg to attach behind the knee. These muscles are more active in fast actions such as running and sprinting whereas the gluteals work better with strong slow movements such as heavy lifts. On the opposite side of the leg to the hamstrings are the *hip flexor* muscles at the front of the thigh bone. These act to pull the thigh bone upwards (flexion of the femur) when you are climbing the stairs for example. Because sitting forms a major part of everyday life, the hip flexor muscles which are shortened in the sitting position are often tight and require stretching rather than strengthening (see p. 77). The *quadriceps* muscles on the front of the thigh straighten and stabilise the knee. The central muscle of the quadriceps group, the *rectus femoris*, also acts over the hip, and so combined hip and knee actions such as those used in squats and lunges, for example, are needed to work it.

The *hip adductors* and *abductors* pull the thigh bone inwards and outwards respectively in a scissor action. They are worked with scissor movements such as the multihip and sitting abductor unit, but will also work during an exercise such as the squat where they will tighten to avoid the leg being pushed into a knock knee or bow leg stance. The lower leg consists of the deep (*soleus*) and surface (*gastrocnemius*) calf muscles, which point the foot and raise the body up onto the toes, and the shin muscle (*tibialis anterior*), which pulls the toes upwards. At the side of the shin we have the *peronei* muscles which pull the foot outwards and help to stabilise the ankle when running.

BREATHING

Look again at the points on p. 107 concerning general weight training practice. With the upper limb movements breathing was timed to breathe out on effort. This is because lifting a weight can increase blood pressure (p. 90) and breathing out will help to minimise this increase. This still applies with lower limb work, especially exercises such as the squat and dead lift where your whole body and the weight are being lifted. However, an additional reason for the breathing order with the upper limb movements is that arm movements will directly influence rib cage movement, helping or hindering chest expansion. With the lower limbs this is obviously not the case, and so the timing of breathing is actually less important. What is important, however, is that you do not hold your breath, but continue to breathe normally throughout the movement.

GENERAL

SQUAT WITH BARBELL FOR FITNESS (SEE ALSO P. 183)

Goal To work all the major lower limb muscles and assist core stability.

Technique Place your feet slightly wider than shoulder width apart and place a light barbell (or powerbar) across your shoulders. Hold the bar (undergrasp) and, keeping your back aligned, bend your knees until your

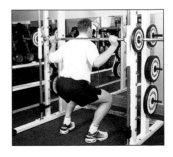

thighs are parallel to the ground. Pause slightly in this lower position and then straighten your legs again to stand up. Breathe normally throughout the movement.

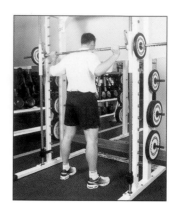

Points to note If you find that your heels lift up as you squat, your calf muscles, achilles tendon, or ankles may be quite inflexible. To reduce the stretch on this area place a small (1–2 cm) block beneath your heels.

LUNGE WITH BARBELL

Goal To work the thigh (quadriceps) and buttock (gluteal) muscles in an alternating single leg action.

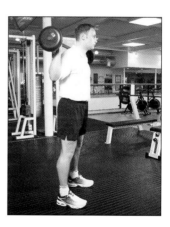

Technique Place a light barbell across your shoulders and stand with your feet shoulder width apart. Step directly forwards with your right foot and lower yourself down onto your left knee. Push yourself back up and repeat the action, stepping with your left foot. Breathe normally throughout the movement.

Points to note As you lunge, the action is to lower the body weight directly downwards rather than forwards. Try to keep your trunk upright rather than angling it from the waist. Your knee should stay over the centre of your foot as you step. If you step too far forwards, your knee remains behind your foot, and if you do not step far enough, your knee will pass over your toes. As you bend your knee it should be more or less level with your leading foot.

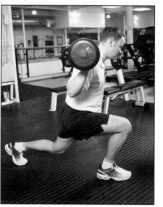

LUNGE WITH DUMB-BELL

Goal To work the thigh (quadriceps) and buttock (gluteal) muscles in an alternating single leg action, with reduced spinal compression.

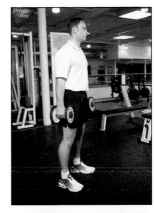

Technique Hold a dumb-bell in each hand and stand with your feet shoulder width apart. Step directly forwards with your right foot and lower yourself down onto your left knee. Push yourself back up and repeat the action, stepping with your left foot. Breathe normally throughout the movement.

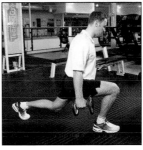

Points to note As you lunge, the action is to lower the body weight directly downwards rather than forwards. Your arms should hang down vertically behind your leading foot rather than in front of it.

LEG PRESS (SEATED)

Goal To work the thigh (quadriceps) muscles, with secondary work on the hip extensors (gluteals and hamstrings).

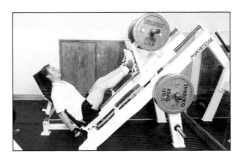

Technique Sit in the leg press machine and adjust the seat position for comfort. Place your feet shoulder width apart and hold on to the machine handles. Exhale and straighten your legs (without locking them rapidly) and then bend them again under control.

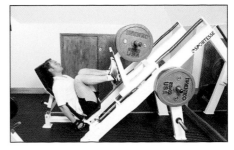

Points to note Placing the feet wider apart allows your knees to pass either side of your chest and increases the available range of motion at the hip. Keeping the feet close together limits hip motion when the knees contact the chest. This movement forces the lower back to bend (flex) and may cause pain if you have a previous back injury. If

LOWER LIMB WEIGHT TRAINING EXERCISES

this is the case, use the dumb-bell lunge (p. 146) or the leg extension (p. 148) instead.

HORIZONTAL LEG PRESS
....

Goal To work all the major leg muscles with reduced spinal loading.

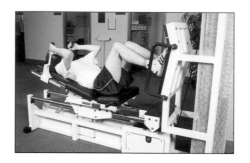

Technique Lie in the leg press unit, placing your shoulders beneath the padded bars and your feet shoulder width apart on the foot plate. Lengthen your spine and tighten your tummy muscles to stabilise your spine. Grasp the machine handles and release the movement, bending your knees to slide the sled downwards towards your feet, inhaling as you do. Stop the motion when your knees are at a 90° bend and then exhale and straighten your legs once more.

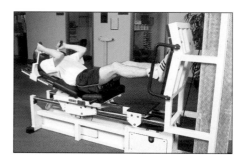

Points to note The knee should pass directly over the centre of the foot as the leg bends. Do not allow the knee to angle inwards (knock knee) or outwards (bow leg).

ISOLATION

LEG EXTENSION
....

Goal To work the thigh (quadriceps) muscles in isolation.

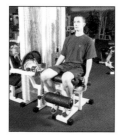

Technique Sit on the leg extension machine and adjust the back rest so that your knee is level with the machine pivot, and adjust the leg roller for comfort. Grip the handles of the machine for stability and straighten your legs. Lock the knees, but do not overstraighten (hyperextend) them. Breathe normally throughout the movement.

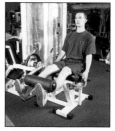

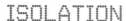

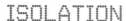

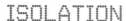

BODYTONING

Points to note As you lock your knees, pulling your feet towards you (ankle dorsiflexion) can help to increase the intensity of the quadriceps contraction.

LEG CURL SEATED

Goal To work the hamstring muscles in isolation, emphasising their action over the knee only.

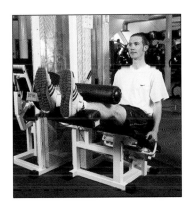

Technique Adjust the machine seat for comfort and hook your calves over the pads. Hold the handles for stability and bend the knees to lift the weight. Allow the knees to straighten again under control. Breathe normally throughout the movement.

Points to note The hamstring muscles work on both the hip and knee, and this exercise only targets knee movement. In addition, this type of movement can also lead to hamstring tightness if performed excessively. Make sure the movement is balanced by performing a hamstring stretching exercise (p. 74) in the same training session. If you have very tight hamstring muscles this exercise is unsuitable for you.

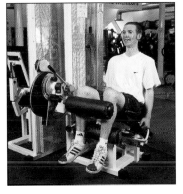

LEG CURL LYING

Goal To work the hamstring muscles in isolation in lying, emphasising their action over the knee only.

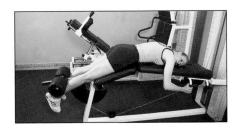

Technique Lie on the leg curl bench with your kneecaps over the bench edge. Hook your heels and lower calves beneath the machine pads and exhale as you bend your knees to raise the weight. Pause in the inner position and then lower the weight under control, inhaling as you do so.

Points to note As with the seated leg curl movement, this exercise can tighten the hamstring muscles and is unsuitable for those with very short hamstrings.

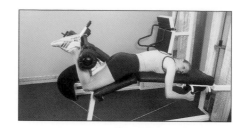

SITTING HIP ADDUCTION

Goal To work the inner hip muscles (adductors) in isolation.

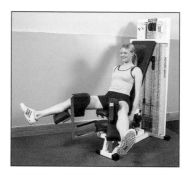

Technique Sit on the adductor machine and adjust the range limiter to suit your degree of flexibility. Place your legs on the machine pads and pull your legs together in a scissor action (hip adduction). Pause in the inner position and then allow the weight to lower under control. Breathe normally throughout the movement.

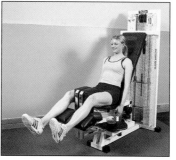

Points to note This exercise will tone and strengthen the hip adductor muscle but also tighten them at the same time. To compensate for this perform adductor stretches (p. 77) in the same workout.

SITTING HIP ABDUCTION

Goal To work the outer hip muscles (abductors) in isolation.

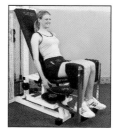

Technique Sit on the abductor machine and adjust the range limiter to suit your degree of flexibility. Place your legs on the machine pads and push your legs apart in a scissor action (hip abduction). Pause in the outer position and then allow the weight to lower under control. Breathe normally throughout the movement.

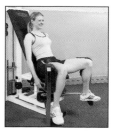

Points to note Some people find this movement awkward because of their degree of hip flexibility in the sitting position. If this is the case, standing hip abduction on a multihip unit is a better alternative.

HIP EXTENSION (GLUT, OR 'TUSH' TONER)

Goal To work the gluteal muscles in isolation.

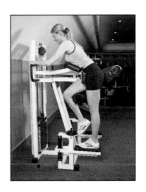

Technique Adjust the machine for your body build and stand with your tummy supported on the machine pad. Hook your right leg beneath the machine pad and lift your bent leg upwards (hip extension), tightening your buttock (gluteal muscles) as you do. Pause in the upper position and then lower under control. Repeat the action with your left leg. Breathe normally throughout the movement.

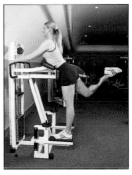

Points to note If you get cramp in your hamstring muscles on the back of your thigh as you perform this action, stretch your hamstrings (p.74) before you perform the exercise.

STRAIGHT LEG CALF RAISE — MACHINE RESISTED

Goal To work the long calf muscle (gastrocnemius).

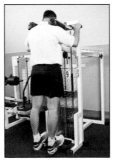
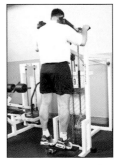

Technique Place the balls of your feet on the machine footplate and position your shoulders under the machine pads. Keeping your legs straight, raise up onto your toes. Pause in the upper position and then lower the weight under control. Allow your heels to move down fully, stretching your calves before you repeat the movement. Breathe normally throughout the movement.

Points to note Altering the foot position (turned in or out) will vary the muscular emphasis of this exercise.

STANDING CALF RAISE WITH DUMB-BELL

Goal To work the long calf muscle (gastrocnemius) one leg at a time.

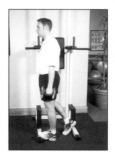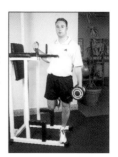

Technique Grasp a dumb-bell in your right hand and hold a machine frame for balance. Place the ball of your right foot on a block, and keeping your legs straight raise up onto your toes. Pause in the upper position and then lower under control. Allow your heel to move down fully, stretching your calf before you repeat the movement on the left leg. Breathe normally throughout the movement.

Points to note Altering the foot position (turned in or out) will vary the muscular emphasis of this exercise.

BENT LEG HEEL RAISE – MACHINE RESISTED

Goal To work the short calf muscle (soleus).

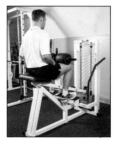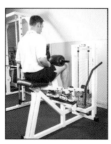

Technique Place the balls of your feet on the machine footplate and position your knees under the machine pads. Keeping your legs bent, raise up onto your toes. Pause in the upper position and then lower the weight under control. Allow your heels to move down fully, stretching your calves before you repeat the movement. Breathe normally throughout the movement.

Points to note Altering the foot position (turned in or out) will vary the muscular emphasis of this exercise.

The trunk has two interacting groups of muscles. For stability the deep abdominals and deep spinal muscles are important. These are covered in the stability section of chapter 7. For movement, the superficial muscles (see Fig. 7.1) are of more importance and these are dealt with in this chapter.

The 'six-pack' muscle is the *rectus abdominis*, two lying on either side of the body joined in the centre. They are divided functionally into two sections, the upper (supra-umbilical) and lower (infra-umbilical) portions. The whole of the muscle works when it contracts, but with a sit-up type action the upper portion is emphasised, and with a leg lift action the lower portion is worked more. The *external oblique* at the side of the trunk has a powerful twisting action, and the portion of this muscle at the side of the body will sideflex the trunk. The *spinal extensor* muscles travel either side of the spine in two thick columns. They will arch (extend) the spine and help to resist bending (rounding) stresses in the spine when lifting.

BREATHING

With both the upper limb and lower limb actions it was important not to hold the breath, but to breathe normally throughout the movements. This was largely to try to minimise the blood pressure changes which can occur in weight training (p. 90), and in the case of the upper limb to link the arm motion to rib cage expansion in breathing. With the trunk, muscle contraction itself is linked to breathing. As we breathe in the diaphragm moves downwards and the tummy (abdominal wall) should move out, bulging. As we breathe out (exhale) the tummy should be drawn in (hollowed) to assist the diaphragm with its job of pushing the air out of the lungs. The general sequence should be to exhale as you tighten the abdominal muscles and inhale as they relax. Do not hold your breath, but continue to breathe throughout the exercise.

BACK EXTENSOR

Goal   To work the back straightening muscles (spinal extensor) muscles, with secondary work on the gluteals (buttocks).

Technique   Adjust the seat and roller of the back extensor for comfort, and fasten the seat-belt. Exhale and tighten your tummy muscles and push backwards, to lift the weight. Hold the inner position and then lower under control.

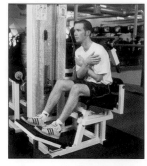

Points to note The position of the pivot point of the machine will alter the effect of this machine. If the pivot is placed at the hip, the action is to tilt the pelvis backwards and extend the spine. With the pivot at the level of the mid lower back (lumbar spine) the pelvis will be more difficult to move but the back will extend further, and arch over the machine roller.

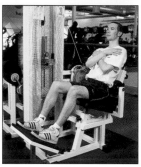

AB CURL MACHINE

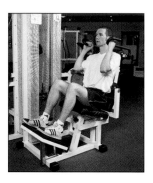

Goal To emphasise work on the central abdominal muscle (rectus abdominis).

Technique Sit on the machine, adjusting the seat height and pads for comfort. Exhale to tighten your abdominal muscles, and bend (flex) your trunk, reaching your head towards your knees, in a curling action. Hold the inner position and then return.

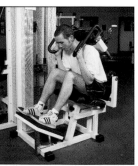

Points to note This movement should be a curling action, keeping the lower spine on the seat back and drawing the rib cage down to the pelvis. This will fully tighten (shorten) the muscle. If you simply lean forwards, allowing your lower spine to leave the seat back, the additional movement has occurred at the hip not the spine.

ROTARY TORSO

Goal   To work the oblique abdominal muscles (internal and external oblique).

Technique   Sit on the machine with your knees blocked against the pads. Rest your forearms on the chest bar and grip the handles. Adjust the range of motion limiter so that it allows you to fully twist your spine but not to overstretch it. Lock the machine and twist to the right and then to the left, lifting the weight as you do so. Make sure that you control the movement in each direction, do not allow the machine to 'run away with you'. Breathe normally throughout the exercise.

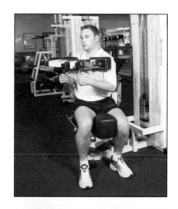

Points to note   The rotary torso action is important as it works the oblique abdominal muscles which are essential to controlled movement of the spine. However, the range of motion limiter must be set correctly to avoid the risk of the machine twisting you too far. For this reason set the limiter to stop the machine movement just short of your full degree of spinal twist (full range motion). In this way you will avoid the possibility of overstretch.

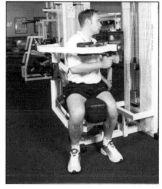

LATERAL FLEXION WITH LOW PULLEY

Goal   To work the trunk side bending muscles (external oblique and quadratus lumborum).

Technique   Stand with your right side facing a low pulley machine and hold the 'D' handle in your right hand. Raise your left hand and place it behind your neck. Side bend (laterally flex) your trunk to the left, reaching your bent elbow towards your knee.

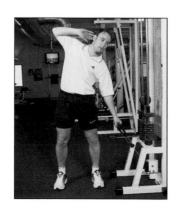

Hold the inner position and then lower the weight under control, bending to the right before you repeat the action. To perform the movement with the other side of the body, hold the 'D' handle in your left hand and bend to the right. Breathe normally throughout the movement.

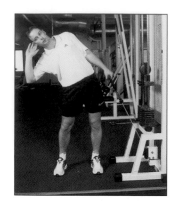

Points to note It is important to fully stretch the muscle by side bending towards the pulley before you side bend away and shorten the muscle.

LATERAL FLEXION WITH DUMB-BELL

Goal To work the trunk side bending muscles (external oblique and quadratus lumborum) with a free weight.

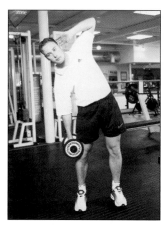

Technique Hold a dumb-bell in your right hand and raise your left hand and place it behind your neck. Side bend (laterally flex) your trunk to the left, reaching your bent elbow towards your knee. Hold the inner position and then lower the weight under control, bending to the right before you repeat the action. Breathe normally throughout the movement. To perform the movement with the other side of the body, hold the dumb-bell handle in your left hand and bend to the right.

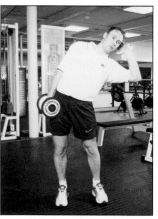

Points to note If you use a dumb-bell in each hand, the two will cancel each other out, the weight on one dumb-bell helping to lift the other. Using one dumb-bell at a time places greater emphasis on the side flexor muscles.

KNEE RAISE – HANGING

Goal To work the lower portion of the abdominal muscles (rectus abdominis and the obliques) together with the hip bending (flexor) muscles.

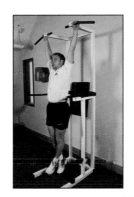

Technique Hold on to a chinning bar with your knees bent, feet resting either on a bench or the floor. Exhale and bend first your knees and hips to bring your legs towards your chest. Finally flex your trunk, pulling your tummy button in. Hold the inner position and then lower under control.

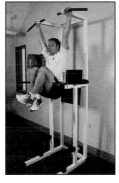

Points to note Try to limit body swing with this movement. Either stop after each repetition and rest your feet on the floor or a gym bench, or ask your training partner to stand behind you to stabilise your body as you lower your legs.

KNEE RAISE – FROM FRAME

Goal To work the lower portion of the abdominal muscles with the hip flexor muscles, using a forearm support position.

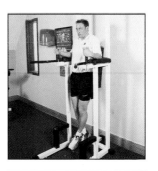

Technique Place your forearms on the machine pads and hold on to the handles. Your feet should rest on a gym bench or the floor. Exhale and bend first your knees and hips to bring your legs towards your chest. Finally flex your trunk pulling your tummy button in. Hold the inner position and then lower under control.

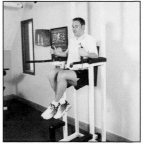

Points to note This action is the same as that of the hanging leg raise, but it reduces the need for grip strength holding a chinning bar.

However, the action can stress the shoulders if they are allowed to raise up or drop too far. Try to maintain the distance between your shoulders and ears throughout the action, lengthening your spine and 'sitting tall' on the frame.

HIP HINGE

Goal To teach the correct bending sequence for the hip and spine.

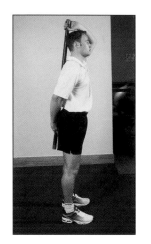

Technique Begin holding a pole along the length of the spine, your right hand reaching overhead to grip the top of the pole, your left hand reaching behind your back to grip the bottom. Place your feet shoulder width apart and unlock your knees. Tighten your tummy muscles and bend forwards keeping your spine straight. Angle from your hips while bending your knees slightly. Stop when your trunk is at a 45° angle and come back to the upright position. Breathe normally throughout the movement.

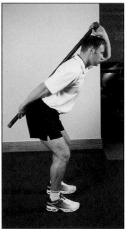

Points to note The pole is a guide to the position of your spine. If you round your spine instead of keeping it straight, the stick will be pushed away from your back. If you hollow your spine, the distance between your lower back and the stick will increase. Aim to maintain the alignment you begin with throughout the movement.

GOOD MORNING

Goal To work the back extensors and buttocks (gluteals) from a functional lifting position.

Technique Before using this exercise, perform the hip hinge movement (above)

BODYTONING

until you are able to maintain spinal alignment easily. Place a light barbell across your shoulders and stand with your feet astride. Keeping your back straight, tighten your tummy muscles and bend your knees slightly. Angle forwards from your hips until your trunk is at 45° to the vertical. Lift back to the starting position and repeat. Breathe normally throughout the movement.

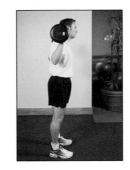

Points to note The aim of this exercise is to maintain spinal alignment and stability as you bend. The amount of weight that is lifted is unimportant. The requirement is for strict technique and accuracy of movement.

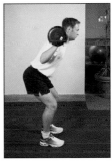

SPINAL EXTENSION

Goal To work the back straightening muscles (spinal extensors) with the buttocks (gluteals).

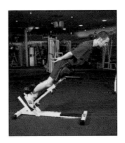

Technique Adjust the machine for comfort and hook your feet or calves under the pads of the machine. Tighten your tummy muscles and lift your body out horizontally keeping your arms by your sides. Hold the position and then slowly lower your trunk and then lift it once more. Breathe normally throughout the movement.

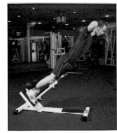

Points to note It is important to tighten the tummy muscles before you lift the trunk. This will help to maintain the alignment of the spine and avoid overhollowing the back (maximum hyperextension).

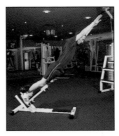

BODYTONING CIRCUITS ❮

PRINCIPLES OF CIRCUIT TRAINING

Weight training programmes are on the whole designed simply to increase strength and muscle tone. If the training aim is to tone up and emphasise cardiovascular (CV) fitness, circuit training can offer a more balanced approach. Circuit training consists of a number of exercises performed in a continuous sequence, with very little rest between each. This type of training emphasises the stamina component of fitness training by keeping the heart rate high and so increasing the amount of aerobic activity.

The circuit can be seen as a structured form of group exercise; a sort of 'regulated aerobics class' that can easily be controlled by an instructor and can be performed in a confined space. Instead of resting after each set, allowing the muscle to recover and letting the heart rate fall, the aim of circuit training is to increase the heart rate and to keep it high. This is achieved by working the various parts of the body in sequence (arms/legs/trunk) without any rest period which allows the heart rate to drop significantly. By alternating muscle groups, local muscle fatigue is avoided, but the continuous activity maintains the workload on the CV system.

DESIGNING GENERAL FITNESS CIRCUITS

A variety of free exercises or apparatus may be used, incorporating different fitness components. Exercises for strength may be interspersed with flexibility, stamina, speed and skill work to give an overall workout. Simple exercises such as push-ups and bent knee sit-ups become more challenging in a circuit format, and specificity of training may be enhanced by mimicking the actions involved in a particular sport. For example, a circuit may be set up on a football pitch involving short sprints, zigzag running, dribbling and shooting skills, in addition to upper body and trunk work.

The circuit may be developed by altering the frequency (number of complete circuits), intensity (resistance, heart rate, range of motion) or duration (number of repetitions) of the various exercises. Either set the number of repetitions, in which case the aim is to complete the circuit as quickly as possible; or specify a time limit with the aim of performing the greatest possible number of repetitions.

ORGANISING THE CIRCUIT

One method of organising the circuit is for each individual to perform a fitness test on the exercises which will comprise the circuit. The individual works to his or her maximum capacity, and the score obtained determines the number of repetitions to be per-

BODYTONING

14

formed during training. In this manner, individuals of various fitness levels are able to train together, each performing the same exercises but at different intensities. In addition, the scores obtained for each exercise may form part of a general fitness evaluation which can be repeated at regular intervals to assess progress. This can be particularly useful in team sports if the first test is performed at the beginning of a season and the repeat evaluations used as a factor in team selection.

The circuit may be set out by sketching each exercise to be performed using 'pin-men' figures, and then writing a brief explanation of each movement beneath. This information is then placed at the relevant exercise station. Large clear figures should be used, and colour coding for easy recognition can be helpful, dividing up the circuit participants into beginners (blue), intermediate (green) and advanced (red). At each station the exercise type or number of repetitions can be represented by a colour, as follows.

Same exercise, but varying number of repetitions	Same number of reps, but different starting positions
Blue 10 reps	Blue Push-up from kneeling
Green 12 reps	Green Standard push-up
Red 15 reps	Red Push up with feet on stool

BODYTONING CIRCUITS FOR SPORT AND INJURY RECOVERY

Circuits can incorporate movements which would normally be carried out as part of a specific sport or work/home activity. This type of training, called a *functional circuit,* is useful for training as it is a task-specific form of training (p. 12) meaning that it exactly matches the performance characteristics of a particular sport. In addition, if used for retraining after injury, the functional circuit can be focused on specific movements that the subject feels weak or at risk. For example, after an ankle injury, walking on an uneven surface (bumpy ground), or after a knee ligament injury, twisting the leg.

The first example is a functional circuit designed for a person recovering from a back injury (see Table 14.1). The aim is to restrengthen the back muscles while avoiding excessive strain on the other back structures. In addition, the circuit encourages good lifting technique and strengthens the legs to enable them to lift more powerfully in day-to-day activities. It is important to liaise with the client's physiotherapist to make sure that the exercises used do not conflict with any treatment programme.

TARGET SPECIFIC CIRCUITS

Targeting specific areas such as bums 'n' tums (see Table 14.2) is also an excellent technique with circuit training. To focus on several exercises for these body areas can be quite monotonous if you are training by yourself. However, the same exercises put in a circuit format can be far more enjoyable and motivating. The group dynamics of a circuit can also spur an individual to work that little bit harder and so increase exercise intensity.

Table 14.1 Circuit for back injury recovery

Exercise	Beginner 40s rest	Intermediate 30s rest	Advanced 20s rest
Warm-up – cycle, sitting upright	3 min	5 min	7 mins
Free squat on to bench	8	10	12
Spinal extension machine	8	10	12
Heel slide (core stability)	12	15	20
Lat pull down	8	10	12
Lunge	8	10	12
Hip hinge action	8	10	12
Seated rowing (machine)	8	10	12

CIRCUIT WEIGHT TRAINING

Instead of using all types of exercise, circuit weight training (CWT) is performed using only resistance training apparatus. In contrast to normal weight training, CWT places less emphasis on heavy overload of a single muscle group, using instead a more general fitness programme. Work on arms, legs and trunk is alternated to prevent fatigue in any one muscle group, but constant activity is maintained so that the heart rate stays high. Various types of work:rest ratio may be used. Typical combinations would be eight

Table 14.2 Circuit for bums 'n' tums

Exercise	Beginner 40s rest	Intermediate 30s rest	Advanced 20s rest
Warm-up – cross trainer, reverse action	2 min	4 min	6 min
Squat	10	12	15
Hip extension machine	8	10	12
Trunk curl	10	12	15
Rotary torso	8	10	12
Lunge	8	10	12
Hip abductor	8	10	12
Dumb-bell side bend	8	10	12
Gymball bridge	8	10	12

or more exercises, with a weight of 40–55 per cent 1RM. As many repetitions as possible should be performed in 30 seconds, for example, with a rest of 15 seconds.

Only small increases in cardio-pulmonary fitness should be expected with this type of training, but CWT has been shown to be particularly effective in helping to maintain fitness and so has an important part to play in rehabilitation. Because of the controlled nature of the activity, it is possible to focus on or to exclude specific parts of the body while still working the rest. This is particularly useful during injury, as general physical condition can be maintained without placing stress on the injured part. For example, if a person has a hamstring injury, specific physiotherapy would be used for the leg, and

CWT could be performed to maintain fitness in the upper body and trunk. Later, a full circuit may be initiated to develop competitive fitness of the whole body.

GENERAL BODYTONING CIRCUIT

This circuit provides three run-throughs of the arms–leg–trunk sequence, with increasing repetitions as fitness improves. Alternatively, the reps may be kept constant and the weight increased. The rest periods between the exercises reduce from 40 seconds to 30 and finally 20 seconds as training progresses. Initially a single circuit is performed three times per week for two weeks, and then two circuits are used three times a week for two weeks. After this period, users may move up to the next category in Table 14.3. Advanced users may increase weight or reps and reduce resting time. Allow a two to three minute recovery period between circuits for 'recovery walking', that is, walking around the gym to maintain the activity but allow a rest period. Finish the training programme with two minutes' stretching as a cool-down.

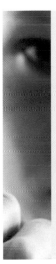

Work/rest periods

In addition to the strength gains expected with a weight training based programme, CWT will increase fitness (measured as maximum oxygen uptake or 'VO2 max'). However, this is only achieved providing the correct work/rest period is used. No fitness changes are seen using 30s work periods and 60s rest, but when a 15s rest period is given, an 11% improvement of fitness is seen (Wilmore *et al.* 1978). Once fitness has been gained (by running, for example) it can be maintained with CWT while strength improves. Following an 8 week programme of running followed by the same length of CWT, fitness gained by the running programme is maintained. In addition, reductions in body fat and strength improvements are also seen (Gettman and Pollock 1981).

BODYTONING CIRCUITS

Table 14.3 General fitness circuit			
Exercise	**Beginner 40s rest**	**Intermediate 30s rest**	**Advanced 20s rest**
Warm-up – cross trainer	3 min	5 min	7 min
Seated chest press	8	10	12
Seated leg press	10	12	15
Rotary torso	8	10	12
Lat pull down	8	10	12
Lunge (stick only, no weight)	10	12	15
Abdominal curl machine	8	10	12
Dumb-bell lateral raise	10	12	15
Hip abductor machine	8	10	12
Spinal extension machine	10	12	15

EXERCISE BANDS ‹

Exercise bands provide an ideal form of portable resistance. They are convenient and inexpensive, and can be used to mimic pulley or spring based exercises at a fraction of the cost. Bands were originally developed for physiotherapy usage from the practice of cutting up car tyre inner tubes to provide resistance for patients performing home exercise. This led to the development of clinical rubber bands and rubber tubing, which then found their way into the fitness market. Use in the fitness market has greatly expanded the variety of equipment available, with handles, foot stirrups, bars and door anchors (used to provide a secure fixation point) now available.

PREPARATION FOR BAND EXERCISE

Before we begin band or tubing exercise there are a number of important safety points to consider. Bands can come loose, slipping from the hand or fixation point, or even breaking. For this reason a client should not look directly at the end of the band as it will strike the eye if released. Turning the head slightly will make it more likely that if released by accident the end of the band will strike the side of the head rather than the eye.

Bands can slip from sweaty hands, so the band should be wound around the hand rather than gripped in the palm. Use approximately 30 cm more band than the length which you require for the range of motion of the movement, to allow for wrapping around the hand.

The band may be secured to the foot using either a purpose-designed foot strap or a figure of eight loop. For the figure of eight loop, the band is passed beneath the foot and then around the ankle/shin, leaving the free end at the level of the heel. By winding the band around both the foot and ankle, it is prevented from either slipping off the foot or sliding up the ankle and rasping the skin as it does so.

Because bands come in rolls, they are powdered to stop the layers of band sticking together. Some clients may have skin allergies which could react to the powder or simply may not like the smell. Tubing has less powder (sometimes none at all) and so is more easily tolerated. In addition, bands are normally made of latex while tubing is normally rubber. Those with latex allergies should either use tubing or latex-free bands which are available at an extra cost.

To reduce the likelihood of the band or tubing breaking, do not stretch it to its maximum degree. The resistance provided by a band is maximal at its full stretch, and proportionally less at shorter extended lengths. If the maximum resistance is required, rather than stretching the band to its limit, simply use a thicker grade band to provide the required resistance, or double the band up.

Because of the nature of rubber, bands and tubing will lose some of their elasticity and become brittle (perished) and more likely to break with time. For this reason bands and tubing should be discarded when they have been used regularly for a six-month period.

Bands must be attached to the body or to external fixation points securely. If bands are tied to an object a secure reef or double knot should be used with at least 20 cm of free band protruding to guard against the knot slipping free. A *toggle* may be used beneath or at the side of a door. This consists of a metal disc (3–4 cm diameter) with a fabric strap attached. The metal disc goes on the other side of the door and the door is firmly closed. The fabric strap protrudes through the gap at the side of the door or beneath it for attachment of the tubing or band. Again the band must be tied to the strap securely. Ensure that the gap between the door and doorframe is not large enough to allow the toggle to slip through, and make sure that the door is closed securely and preferably locked to prevent the toggle from slipping. Safety factors are summarised in Table 15.1.

Table 15.1 Safety factors when using exercise bands and tubing
• Do not look at the end of the band, turn your head away slightly.   • Wind the band around the hand a number of times to stop it slipping, and use a figure of eight loop over the foot.   • Tubing has less powder coating on it than bands, so use tubing if the client does not like the powder.   • If a client has a latex allergy use latex-free bands or rubber tubing instead.   • Do not stretch a band/tubing to its fullest extent.   • Discard bands/tubing when they begin to lose their elasticity.   • Make sure bands are attached to objects securely – use a toggle.

BREATHING

Because band exercises involve resistance the timing of breathing is important. When a muscle contracts it squeezes the blood vessels travelling through it, increasing blood pressure. With large muscles such as those of the legs and chest, this rise in blood pressure can be significant. Holding the breath will also increase blood pressure because the lungs will press on the large vessels travelling from the heart. The combination of resistance training and holding the breath could therefore produce increases in blood pressure which may be quite serious for seniors, unfit individuals and those with heart or circulatory problems. To minimise this, breathe out as you stretch the bands to help keep the blood pressure more normal, if you are using heavy resistances. For light resistances you should simply breathe normally throughout the movement, and not hold your breath.

BENCH PRESS (BAND ACROSS SHOULDERS)

Goal To strengthen the pushing muscles of the chest (pectorals) and arms (triceps).

Technique Lie on a gym bench with a band passing behind your shoulders. Hold the ends of the band in each hand. The action is to push (press) the arms out straight either together or individually. Hold the extended position and then allow the arm to bend again under control.

Points to note The exercise can also be performed lying on the floor or standing against a wall. In both cases the range of motion is reduced because the elbow is not able to move backwards as far as it does when you are on a gym bench.

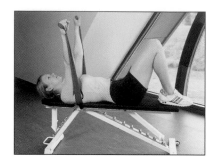

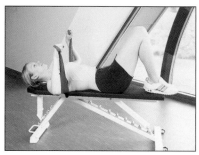

SHOULDER ABDUCTION

Goal Stand with a band passing beneath your feet, with the ends held in each hand.

Technique Keeping your arms locked at the elbow, take your arms out to the side (shoulder abduction) either as far as the horizontal, or fully overhead, and then slowly lower them back to the side of your body. As you move the arm, slightly twist it so that the knuckles face first upwards to the ceiling and then backwards to the wall behind you (lateral rotation of the shoulder joint).

Points to note As the arm moves sideways into abduction, there is a risk of trapping structures between the moving arm bone and the bony roof of the joint (acromion process). Laterally rotating the

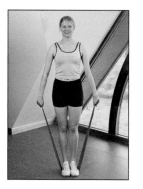

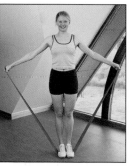

arm by turning it outwards reduces the likelihood of this happening. In addition, stopping the action at the horizontal position and then lowering also minimises the risk of trapping.

STANDING ARM EXTENSION

Goal To tone the muscle on the back of the arm (triceps).

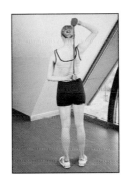

Technique Hold the ends of a band in each hand. Pass the band over the back of the shoulder and hold one arm across your lower back with the other overhead. Begin with your overhead arm bent (elbow flexed) and the slack taken up from the band. The action is to straighten the upper arm overhead while fixing the lower end of the band with the hand of the lower arm.

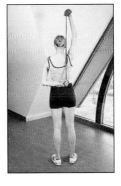

Points to note As you reach overhead there is a tendency to allow the elbow to move outwards. This alters the line of pull of the triceps muscle and reduces the effectiveness of the exercise. Aim to keep the elbow tucked into the side of the head throughout the movement.

ARM CURL

Goal To strengthen the arm flexor muscles (biceps and brachialis) while maintaining whole body alignment.

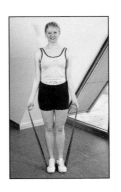
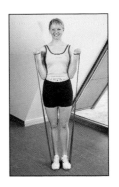

Technique Begin with your feet slightly more than shoulder width apart. Pass a band beneath your feet and grip the ends in each hand. Slightly soften (bend) the knees and stabilise the shoulders (see p. 44), lengthening the spine as you do so. Bend the arms and then allow them to straighten under control. For a single arm curl action, pass the band under one foot only, and grip the band ends in the hand on the same side of the body.

Points to note   You can achieve a slightly different muscle effect by leading the movement with your hand placed thumb upwards (midway between pronation and supination). This will increase the emphasis on the brachioradialis muscle of the forearm.

SHOULDER ROTATION WITH ELBOW SUPPORT

Goal To strengthen the rotator cuff muscles of the shoulder in the abducted position.

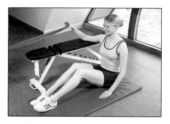

Technique   Sit on the floor with your upper arm at 90° to your body and your fore-arm vertical, hand pointing to the ceiling. Support your upper arm on a bench. Fix a band either behind you (medial rotation) or in front of you (lateral rotation) and turn your arm so that your hand moves closer to the bench top. Restrict the movement to your shoulder, keeping a constant 90° angle at your elbow.

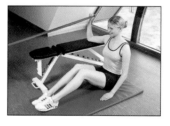

Points to note   This action works the rotator cuff muscles with the arm in a functionally abducted position. However, with the arm in line with the chest, there is more chance of trapping structures within the shoulder joint (a condition called 'impingement'). To avoid this, bring the elbow forward so that the upper arm is at a 30° angle to the line of your back.

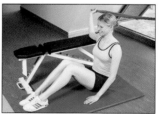

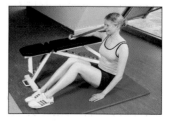

LATERAL SHOULDER ROTATION (FREE STANDING)

Goal To strengthen the rotator cuff muscles of the shoulder, while reducing the abduction range required at the shoulder joint.

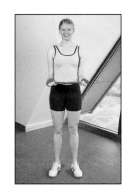

Technique Keep the upper arms at your sides, elbows tucked in and bend your elbows to 90°. Hold the ends of a band in each hand, and stretch the band by twisting the upper arms from the shoulders. The forearms should move as though sliding over a table top, staying on the horizontal.

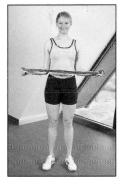

Points to note Many people have a limited range of outward turning (lateral rotation) at the shoulder, and this can be an important factor in some types of shoulder pain. This exercise will both strengthen the lateral rotator muscles, and increase the amount of movement.

SCAPULAR STABILISATION

Goal To re-educate the movement of scapular stabilisation and redevelop the stabilising muscles.

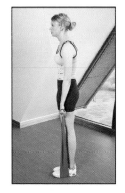

Technique Begin with a band placed beneath your feet, each end held in your hands. Wind the band around the hands to tighten it sufficiently to give you a feeling of your shoulder blades being pulled down gently. Allow your shoulders to be pulled both back and downwards, and maintain this position for 10–20 seconds.

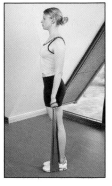

Points to note Many people have very tight muscles around the neck and shoulders. They will often feel a stretch in the upper part of the trapezius muscle which travels from the top of the shoulder to the neck and base of the skull. Over time this muscle will stretch out using this exercise, and the tension will reduce.

STANDING SQUAT

Goal To strengthen the thigh (quadriceps) and bottom (gluteal) muscles at the same time.

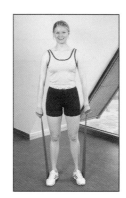

Technique Begin standing on a band with your feet slightly more than shoulder width apart. Grasp the ends of the band in each hand pulling the band tighter. Bend the hips and knees into a squat position, keeping the back straight and upright. Maintain this low position for one second and then stand up again.

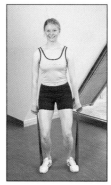

Points to note The power for the exercise must come from the legs only. Keep the arms straight and inactive throughout the movement, avoiding the temptation to pull up with the arms.

SITTING LEG PRESS

Goal To strengthen the front and back thigh muscles (quadriceps and hamstrings) simultaneously.

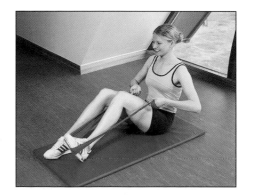

Technique Sit on the floor with your knees bent. Hold both ends of a band in one hand and loop the band around the foot of one leg. Lift the heel of this foot off the floor slightly and extend the leg using a straight pressing action. Pause in the straight position and then allow the leg to flex slowly under control.

BODY TONING

Points to note As the knee extends, it should lock out but not *hyerpextend*, that is, bend back on itself. If you find your knees do this, place a small folded towel behind the knee on the floor. As the knee extends, the towel will block the back of the knee and prevent the excessive backward bend.

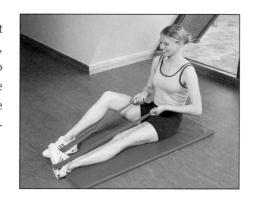

LEG EXTENSION ON CHAIR

Goal Begin sitting on a firm dining chair or gym bench, and tie one end of the band on to the chair leg. Loop the other end over your foot using a figure of eight (or use a foot stirrup).

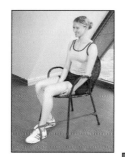

Technique Straighten the leg, hold it straight for 3–5 seconds and then lower slowly.

Points to note As you lock the knee out, do not allow it to 'snap back', but lock it gradually. Snapping the knee back can over-stretch and damage the structures at the back of the knee (popliteal structures).

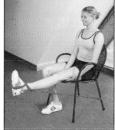

HIP ADDUCTION

Goal To strengthen the hip adductor muscles on the inside of the thigh.

Technique Begin sitting on the floor with your legs apart, in a scissor action (hip abduction). Fasten a band around one leg and attach the end of the band to a secure fixation point, on the outside of the knee. Bring the leg inwards towards the other leg (hip adduction). Hold the inner position for

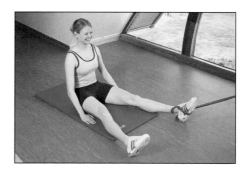

2–3 seconds against the resistance of the band and then allow the leg to move out again under control. Repeat the movement with the other leg.

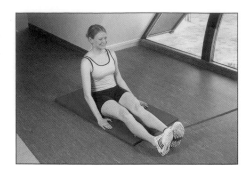

Points to note   If you use a heavy resistance band, there is a tendency to slip on the ground. To prevent this, bend the other leg and place the foot flat on the floor to aid grip.

LYING HAMSTRING STRETCH

Goal   To stretch the hamstring muscles using a neuromuscular technique.

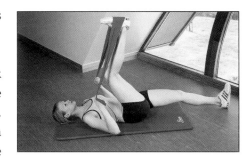

Technique   Lie on the floor on your back with both legs straight. Bend one knee to the chest and hook a band beneath your foot. Use your thigh muscles (quadriceps) to begin straightening your leg and at the same time to stretch your hamstring muscles on the back of the thigh.

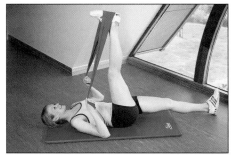

Points to note   When one muscle is worked (contracts) the muscle on the opposite side of the limb will relax through a natural reflex mechanism called *reciprocal innervation*. This exercise uses this reflex to enable you to stretch your hamstrings further than would otherwise be possible.

LYING TRUNK ROTATION (BAND FIXED)

Goal   To strengthen the trunk rotator muscles (oblique abdominals).

Technique   Begin lying on the floor with one leg bent at the knee and hip. Fasten a band around the bent knee and attach the end of the band to a secure fixation point, on the outside of the knee. Twist the spine and turn the whole leg inwards bringing the bent knee across the straight leg to the floor. Pause in this lower position and then draw the leg back to the starting position. Perform the same movement with the band attached to the other leg.

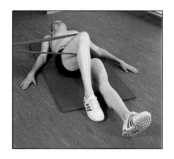

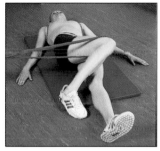

Points to note As the spine twists, the hip on the side of the bent knee will lift from the ground. This is fine, but do not allow the trunk to lift as well. Keep the shoulders and chest fixed to the ground and limit the movement to the spine itself.

RESISTED WALKING/JOGGING

Goal To strengthen the leg muscles and aid balance and muscle reaction speed.

Technique Pass a band around your waist and attach the end of the band to a secure fixation point behind you at waist level or get your training partner to hold the band. Step forwards to tighten the band and maintain this tightness throughout the exercise. Begin walking on the spot, gradually bringing the knees higher and speeding the action up. Progress to gentle jogging on the spot and eventually faster jogging using a high knee raise.

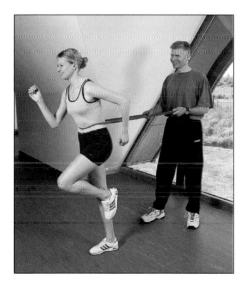

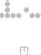

Points to note Because the band is pulling you back, your balance will be aided by leaning forwards slightly. Make sure as you perform the movement that you do not 'hammer' the feet into the ground. As you land, place the toes and then the heels on the ground, taking your weight through your whole foot. Do not stay up on your toes.

STABILITY BALL ‹

The stability ball offers a number of different exercises which can be used to increase the variety of a bodytoning programme. It is one of a number of pieces of equipment which works on balance and coordination as well as strength and tone. Stability balls really come into their own for core stability training, challenging the trunk stabilising muscles in all movement directions, a feature called *multidirectional stability*.

Pick a stability ball which is the correct size for you. You should be comfortable when you sit on it and your hips and knees should be at a 90° bend when sitting upright. If you are new to using the ball perform the 'gymball introduction' before progressing to further movements as it is designed to improve balance on the ball and make usage safer.

GYMBALL INTRODUCTION

Begin with the ball positioned next to a gym bench (or secure dining chair at home). Place one hand on the bench for balance and sit upright on the ball. Begin by rocking from one buttock to the other five times and then leaning slightly forwards and backwards five times. Repeat these movements with your hands off the bench but remaining slightly above it and then finally with your arms out to the side in a 'T' shape. Only when you are confident with your balance should you move away from the bench. If you are on a polished studio floor, place the ball on a 'collar' (circle of plastic), or a folded towel to stop it slipping.

The next exercise is called gymball walking. Sit upright with your feet flat on the floor. Lift one heel (keeping the toes on the ground), place it back on the ground and then lift the other. Perform this movement alternately ten times. Progress to lifting the whole foot and leg from the ground by 5–10 cm, again alternating legs. Finally, straighten one leg out fully and hold this single leg position for 5–10 seconds. When you are confident doing this and you do not wobble too much, reach your arms overhead ten times (still on one leg). Once you have reached this stage your balance on the gymball has improved sufficiently to move on to the specific gymball exercises.

BODYTONING

16

ABDOMINAL SLIDE

Goal Controlling the action of the central abdominal muscle (rectus abdominis) while moving.

Technique Begin sitting on the ball with your knees shoulder width apart and feet flat on the floor. Hollow the abdominal muscles to flatten the contour of the stomach. This flat contour should be maintained throughout the action, avoiding a 'domed' appearance of the abdominal wall. Tilt the pelvis backwards to flatten the back. Continue this movement to curl (flex) the trunk so that the tailbone (sacrum) and then the lower (lumbar) spine and eventually the upper (thoracic) spine rest on the ball. In the end position the ball rests between the shoulder blades and you look over the top of your knees. Maintain the tightness in the abdominal muscles but breathe normally. Do not hold your breath.

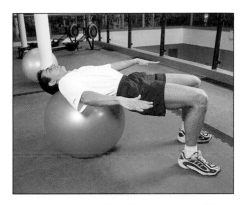

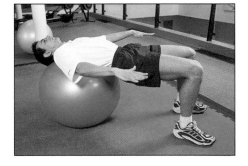

Points to note Make sure that the ball remains in the centre of the back as you move, so that it does not go to the side forcing you to slip off the ball. Reaching your hands out and forwards aids the general balance and control of the movement.

HALF SITTING ARM AND LEG MOVEMENTS

Goal Maintaining core stability and trunk alignment while moving the arms and legs.

Technique Perform the abdominal slide action as described above and hold the final position with the abdominal wall flat and trunk curled. Straighten one leg, maintaining balance on the ball, and then place the

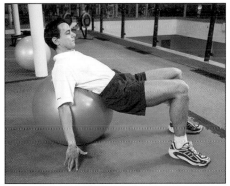

foot back on the ground. Straighten the opposite leg and repeat this movement alternatively maintaining the lumbar position.

With the feet flat on the ground, reach one arm towards the ceiling and bring it back to the waist and then the second arm towards the ceiling. Alternate this movement.

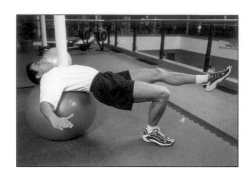

Finally, perform the alternating leg and alternating arm movements at the same time, straightening the right leg and reaching overhead with the left arm. Go back to the rest position and then straighten the left leg and right arm overhead.

Points to note   Because this exercise involves quite advanced coordination, spend some time working just with the legs and then just with the arms before putting both arms and legs together.

LYING TRUNK CURL OVER BALL

Goal   Strengthens the upper part of the abdominal muscles (rectus abdominus) through its full movement range.

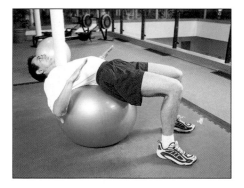

Technique   Begin lying over the ball with your feet wide (one and a half shoulder widths) apart, and flat on the floor. Start with the ball resting on your lower and middle spine, and allow your trunk to extend over the ball so that you look back towards the floor. Breathe out and tighten your abdominal muscles. Initiate the movement by bending your head to place your chin on your chest and then bend your trunk from the top to the bottom to look towards your knees. Hold this position for 2 seconds and then slowly release the movement, allowing the trunk to extend. The head should be the final part of the body to move.

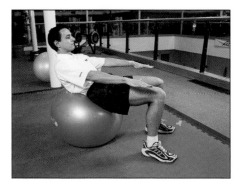

Points to note This movement produces full range motion of the lumbar spine but must be controlled. Taller individuals who have longer spines are likely to find the action harder due to the leverage effects. If you find the movement difficult to control, reduce the range of motion and perform the trunk curl movement without spinal extension. The action is one of trunk *curling* rather than trunk *lifting*. As you round the spine, move it segment by segment, not as a whole unit.

LYING TRUNK CURL WITH LEG LEFT

Goal Strengthens the upper and lower part of the central abdominal muscle (rectus abdominus).

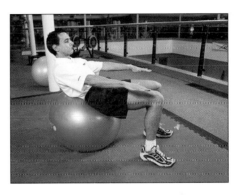

Technique Perform the lying trunk curl as described above. Move into the inner range position with the trunk flexed, looking towards your knee, and maintain this position. Lift one leg, straightening the knee, hold this position breathing normally and then lower. Move first the leg until the foot is flat on the floor and then the trunk back into extension. Repeat the movement, this time lifting the left leg.

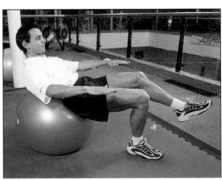

Points to note By lifting the leg in this exercise, the lower portion of the abdominal muscles are further challenged. In addition because only one foot is now on the floor, the balance requirements have been increased. This movement, therefore, both strengthens the trunk muscles and enhances general whole body balance.

SUPERMAN

Goal To strengthen and enhance the endurance of the spinal extensor muscles and the gluteals.

Technique Begin with the ball placed close to a wall. Lie on your front with your abdomen over the ball, and your hands flat on the floor in a press-up position. Your legs should be apart and your feet flat against the wall. Tighten your abdominal muscles and brace your legs until you are completely straight. Lift first one and then the other arm towards your sides and brace your shoulders. Maintain this position for the count of three, breathing normally, and then place your arms back on the floor.

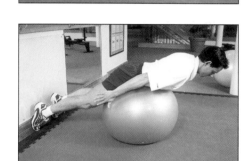

Points to note If you find it difficult to hold your feet flat on to the wall, work with a training partner and get them to steady your legs while you lift until such time as you are confident with the technique of this movement.

SUPERMAN WITH ARMS

Goal To build endurance in the spinal extensor muscles and the gluteals, and also to work the shoulder retractors.

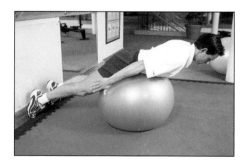

Technique Perform the basic superman movement as above. When you lift one arm, instead of taking it back towards your side, reach it forwards above your head towards the horizontal. Hold this position then lower the arm, lift the opposite arm and maintain the position. Once you are comfortable with this position, progress to lifting first one and then the other arm until both are reaching forwards to the horizontal. Maintain this position for 3 seconds, breathing normally.

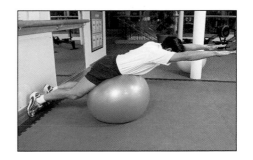

Points to note You should aim to straighten your arms so that they become level with your shoulders. However, if you lack shoulder flexibility, and find this uncomfortable, reach your arms as far forwards as is comfortable for your degree of flexibility.

BRIDGING

Goal To tone the gluteal muscles and spinal extensors.

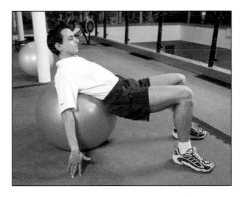

Technique Begin the exercise sitting on the floor with your feet shoulder width apart and flat on the floor. Your shoulders rest on the gymball and your hands are on the floor. Breath out and tighten your abdominal muscles and buttocks and lift your pelvis until your shoulders, hips and knees are in line. Take first one arm and then the other off the ground and place your arms by your sides. Hold the position for a count of three and then slowly lower.

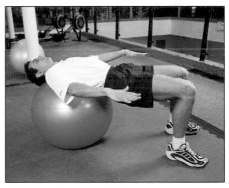

If you find it difficult to lift up into this position, begin with your shoulders on the gymball and your hips on a gym bench. Initially, tighten your abdominal muscles and your gluteal muscles to lift your buttocks 5 or 10 cm from the bench, holding the bridge position. Once you are confident with this movement, have your training partner slide the bench away when you are in the bridge position and lower down to the floor under control.

Points to note Part of the work of this exercise is moving into the position using concentric activity and part is actually holding the position using isometric activity. Rather than increasing the number of repetitions, build up the holding time of the bridge exercise itself. Begin by holding for 3 to 5 seconds and progress the holding until you can maintain the bridge for 20 to 30 seconds breathing normally.

BRIDGE WITH LEG LIFT

Goal To strengthen the upper and lower abdominals while increasing stability control.

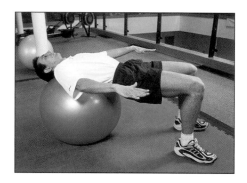

Technique Begin in the bridge position as before, maintain the bridge for 3 seconds and then lift the right leg towards the horizontal. Maintain this position for 2 to 3 seconds, lower the right leg, then lift the left.

Points to note This exercise increases the overload of the movement in terms of muscle work but also in terms of balance and coordination. This latter aspect can be further increased by asking a training partner to gently push against your hips from side to side, increasing the sideways displacement. Your aim is to try to resist their pressure.

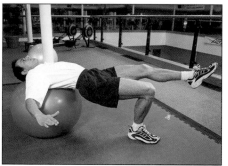

REVERSE BRIDGE

Goal To strengthen the trunk and hip muscles simultaneously.

Technique Begin lying on the floor on a mat with your arms at 45° to your trunk. Place your calf muscles on the stability ball, and tighten your abdominal muscles. Press your calves down into the gymball to lift your hips upwards. Aim to align your shoulders, hips and knees into a straight line.

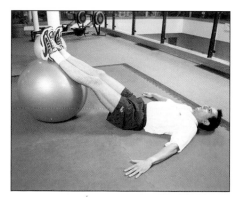

Maintain the position for 3 seconds, breathing normally, then lower.

Points to note This exercise works the backside muscles (gluteals) quite hard in addition to the trunk muscles. To increase the overload on the gluteal muscles, place one leg in the centre of the ball and lift the opposite leg so you are pressing your full body weight into the ball with a *single leg* only. A further modification is the *heel bridge*. This begins as the reverse bridge, but this time simply place your heels on the ball rather than your calf muscles. This increases the overload of the movement as more of your body is off the floor.

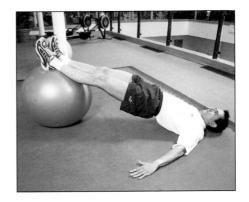

PRONE-FALL

Goal Provides contraction of the hip and trunk muscles together.

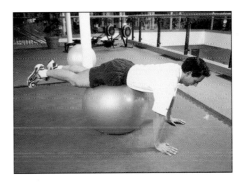

Technique Begin in a press-up position with a gymball placed beneath your thighs. Your legs should be together, hands flat on the floor. Keeping your alignment, walk your hands forwards so that the ball moves down your legs towards your knees and finally your shins. Maintain this position and then walk backwards so that the ball moves back again towards your waist. Breathe normally throughout the movement. Do not hold your breath.

Points to note A sideways movement may also be used, rocking the ball from side to side to work the oblique abdominal muscles and the trunk side flexors.

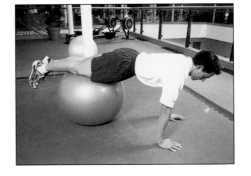

PRONE FALL WITH SINGLE LEG LIFT

Goal Increase the overload of the gluteal muscles in the prone fall action.

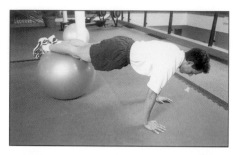

Technique Begin in the starting position of the prone fall action described above. This time, instead of walking the hands forwards, breathe out and tighten the abdominal and gluteal muscles, and lift one leg. Hold the position for between 3 and 5 seconds breathing normally, lower the leg and then lift the opposite leg.

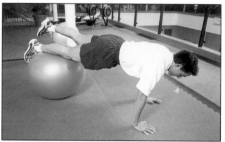

Points to note The single leg which remains on the ball must stay in the centre of the ball for more stability. If the leg is placed off centre on the ball, the ball may slide sideways.

DOUBLE LEG RAISE

Goal To work the gluteal muscles intensely.

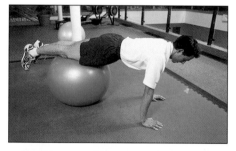

Technique Beginning in the prone fall position described above, walk the hands backwards until the ball is beneath your waist and the legs are unsupported. Maintain this position with both legs aligned along the horizontal for between 3 and 5 seconds breathing normally. Do not hold your breath.

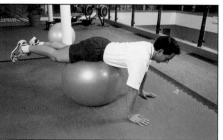

Points to note Because this is an intense movement, there is a tendency to hyperextend the lumbar spine. This can create dangerous compression forces in the spinal joints and must be avoided. Tightening the abdominal muscles and maintaining their contraction throughout the leg raise will help to protect the spine.

Weight lifting exercises can be used in bodytoning and often provide a whole body workout, taxing the arms, legs and trunk simultaneously. The balance and coordination involved in the movements provide an additional angle to your workout, emphasising skill as well as strength. Because the actions involve skill, initially little weight should be used until the technique of the movement has been learnt well. The most important factor when performing the lifts is body alignment. The back must be kept in its neutral position whenever possible (see p. 43), and the legs kept aligned with the knee passing over the centre of the foot. Avoid knock knee or bow leg positions as they stress the ligaments at the side of the knee.

SQUAT (SEE ALSO P. 145)

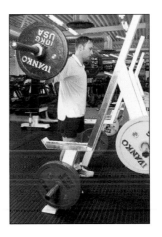

Goal To work all the leg muscles together, with secondary work on the trunk.

Technique Begin the movement with the feet slightly wider than shoulder width apart and the feet turned out slightly. The bar lies across the shoulders (pad the bar if it digs into you). Hold the bar for balance and tighten your tummy muscles. Fix your eyes on a distant object to aid balance and bend your knees to lower your body. As your knees bend, aim to pass your knee directly over the centre of your foot. Stop when your thigh is parallel to the ground and then straighten the legs to push yourself up again. Pause before repeating the movement.

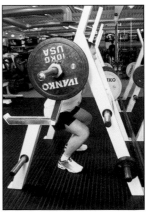

Points to note A number of faults can occur in the squat as outlined in Table 17.1. The squat movement can also be performed with the bar across the front of the shoulders and chest (*front squat*), with the arms folded and elbows level with the shoulders. Holding the bar behind you just under the buttocks (*hack squat*) is another alternative. The hack squat has the advantage that it takes the weight off the shoulders and back and places it closer to the centre of the body.

Table 17.1 Common errors when performing a squat

Error	Technique modification
Knees move inwards (knock knee)	Foot may be flattening too much (pronation). Wear more supporting shoes and practise the movement in front of a mirror. Aim to keep the knee over the foot.
Knees stay behind feet throughout movement	Ankle forward bending (dorsiflexion) may be limited. Place a 1–2cms wooden block beneath the heels. Squat onto a bench without a weight and practise pressing the knee forwards.
Back angles too far forward	Keep the spine more verticle and monitor your posture by standing side on to a mirror.
Spine flexes between the shoulders (thoracic region)	Press the breastbone (sternum) forwards and draw the shoulder blades (scapulae) down and in using a bracing action.
Low back hollows excessively (increased lumbar lordosis)	Tighten the abdominal muscles and hold them tight throughout the movement. Practise hip flexor muscle stretching (page 77).
Heel lift	Position your weight over the centre of your foot rather than through your toes. Check your ankle flexibility and use a wooden block beneath your heals if your ankle forward bend is tight.
Bar dips to one side	Practise the squat in front of a mirror and use a horizontal line drawn on the mirror to line up the bar.
Bouncing in the low position	Practise squatting onto a bench and gradually lower the weight into the final position.

HANG CLEAN

Goal To provide high intensity work to the legs and trunk.

Technique Hold a powerbar or light barbell on your thighs at arm's length. Bend your knees and lean forwards slightly. In a single rapid action, straighten your knees and pull the bar upwards towards your chest, lifting right up onto your toes. As the bar reaches chest level, bend your knees and dip under the bar, resting it across your upper chest and shoulders. Bend the knees once again to lower the bar under control.

Points to note This action depends on timing. The legs provide the power and momentum to the bar. As it travels upwards through its own impetus, you dip under it at the top of its movement. Practise the movement with a stick (broom handle) before you use a weight.

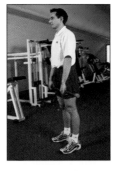
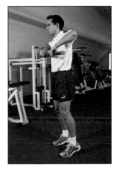
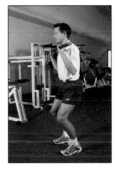
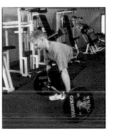

POWER CLEAN

Goal To provide high intensity work to the legs and trunk through greater range.

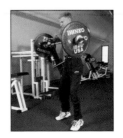
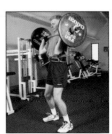

Technique Stand behind a barbell with your feet shoulder width apart. Your shins should be 10–15 cm behind the bar. Tighten your tummy muscles and bend your knees to squat down and grip the bar (overgrasp). Straighten your legs and pull the bar directly upwards on a vertical path. Allow the momentum of the bar to carry it upwards to chest level and, as it begins to slow down, bend your knees and dip beneath the bar to rest it on the top of the chest and shoulders.

Points to note If you find this exercise difficult to control, begin with the bar resting on a bench to bring it above ground level.

CLEAN AND JERK

Goal To coordinate the leg, trunk and arm muscles into a single explosive action.

Technique Take up a squat position, holding a stick or powerbar 20–30 cm above the ground with your feet shoulder width apart. Tighten your tummy muscles and straighten your legs to pull the bar directly upwards on a vertical path. Allow the momentum of the bar to carry it upwards to chest level and, as it begins to slow down, bend your knees and dip beneath the bar to rest it on the top of the chest and shoulders. From this position lift the bar overhead by throwing your legs into a lunge position with one foot forwards and one back, and dipping beneath the bar as you straighten your arms to press the bar upwards.

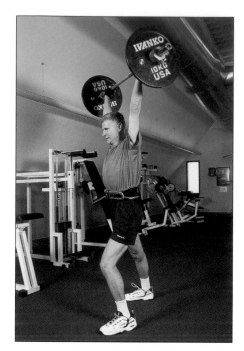

Points to note This is a complex exercise which should only be attempted with a barbell if you are supervised by a qualified instructor.

POWER PRESS (PUSH PRESS)

Goal To provide high intensity work to the shoulders and arms.

Technique Stand with a powerbar or light barbell across your upper chest and shoulders, holding the bar wider than shoulder width apart. Dip your knees and then rapidly straighten them, raising up onto your toes. At the same time, straighten the arms to press the bar overhead. Lower the weight under control, sinking down through your knees as the bar approaches your upper chest. You may use a lunge stance to improve your balance.

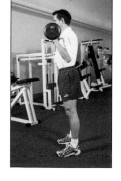
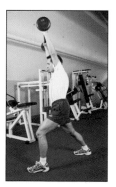

Points to note This action allows a larger weight to be lifted than with a standard shoulder pressing action. Lower the weight slowly to emphasise the eccentric component of the action. The movement may also be performed beginning with the weight across the shoulders to press the bar behind the neck.

DEAD LIFT

Goal To work the leg, hip and trunk muscles in a functional lifting pattern.

Technique Stand behind a barbell with your feet shoulder width apart. Your shins should be 10–15 cm behind the bar. Tighten your tummy muscles and bend your knees to squat down and grip the bar (overgrasp). Straighten your legs and pull the bar directly upwards on a vertical path. Pause in the upward position and then lower the weight, bending the knees and keeping the back straight.

Points to note Keep the hips low on this movement. If the hips initiate the movement rather than the shoulders, the back will bend. The bar must move close to the legs throughout the movement. Table 17.2 shows common errors which may occur in the dead lift.

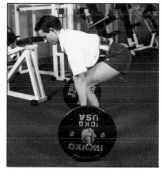

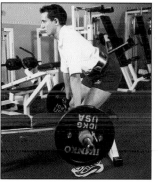

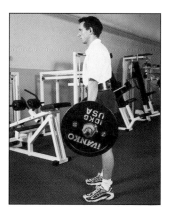

Table 17.2 Common errors when performing a dead lift	
Error	**Technique modification**
Back angle too far forwards	Begin the movement by pressing the shoulders back and leaning backwards slightly.
Back bends	Press your breastbone (sternum) outwards and draw your shoulder blades down and in (bracing) at the beginning of the movement before you move the bar.
Bar hits knee	Straighten knees slightly before you lift the bar from the ground.
Bar bounces on floor	Use a lighter weight and control its descent as you place the bar on the floor. Excessive bar bouncing can increase the loading forces on the spine.
Bar slips from hands	Use a mixed grip with one hand overgrasp and the other undergrasp. Alternate the hand positions throughout your workout.
Knees lock out painfully	Slow the end of the movement down and do not press the knees backwards as you stand up.
User experiences elbow or shoulder pain	Keep the arms locked throughout the movement and do not shrug the shoulders.

DUMB-BELL JUMP SQUAT

Goal To provide a rapid overload on the leg muscles to build jumping power.

Technique Hold a light dumb-bell in each hand. Bend the knees and angle the trunk forwards into a squat position. Rapidly jump upwards, keeping your arms straight. As you land, sink down on your knees to absorb the shock of landing and repeat the action.

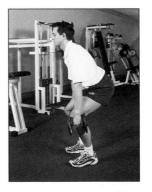

Points to note The upward movement of this exercise is a rapid jump, but the downward movement is slower and controlled. The result should be a silent landing. If you hear your feet stamping on the ground, you are landing too hard. Make sure you land through the foot and knee, softening (flexing) the ankle, knee and hip as you strike the ground.

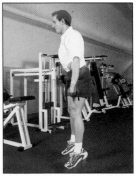

In the gym, there is often an emphasis on movements being slow and controlled. This is laudable from a safety perspective, but many movements in sport and everyday life are performed quickly, with sudden bursts of speed and rapid alteration of movement. Often movements are unexpected, taking you by surprise, and the ability of the body to cope with these changes is vital. If this is what sport and general life present, our training must prepare us for this, and that is the function of this chapter.

THE PHYSIOLOGY OF MUSCLE SPEED

When a movement is performed rapidly, extra force is developed. Try throwing a ball slowly and you will notice that it does not go very far. Throw it quickly and the ball goes much further because you have developed extra force to propel it through the air. Where does this extra force come from? We saw in chapter 3 that muscles contract (pull) when a nerve impulse causes muscle filaments to move together. The muscle filaments, called *actin* and *myosin*, are surrounded by membranes which hold the muscle together. However, these same membranes are also elastic and, when a muscle is stretched, they will recoil a little like a giant elastic band. Take a bench press action (p. 109): if the bar is resting on the chest, to push it up our chest muscles pull on the arms to straighten them. To gain extra force, however, we can begin the movement with the arms straight. As we lower the weight onto the chest, the chest muscles are now stretched first. As we come to lift the weight we have the force from the contracting muscle plus the force created by elastic recoil. The two together give a greater total force. This type of contraction which involves stretching before contraction of the muscle is known as *pre-stretching* and is an important component of speed training.

When we looked at stretching (p. 26) we saw that the muscle was controlled by a number of reflexes. When we stretch a muscle suddenly, it tightens up to protect itself by trying to withstand the stretching force. This process is called the *stretch reflex*, and is the third important part of speed training. If, when we begin our bench press movement, we lower the weight onto the chest rapidly (controlling its fall), in addition to the elastic recoil of the muscle described above, the stretch reflex comes in to play. We now have a third factor to increase the muscle force. In rapid movements then we have force from three areas – normal muscle contraction, elastic recoil and the muscle reflexes. All three combined give us the rapid springing actions we need for jumping, throwing and kicking (see Table 18.1).

To be able to use these three components of muscle force, speed training activities have to be fast, and they have to begin with pre-stretching; that is, the muscle must be

BODYTONING FOR SPEED

stretched just before it is contracted to 'wind it up'. This is similar to taking your arm back before you throw, or bending your knees before you jump upwards. Training which uses these types of actions is called *plyometrics*. When we use speed training to work against our body weight or the weight of a light powerbar or medicine ball, for example, something more is happening. Not only are we moving quickly (*speed*) but we are moving quickly against a resistance. This extra angle changes speed to *power*. We are now moving quickly and working even harder to do so.

Table 18.1 Muscle force for speed training	
MUSCLE CONTRACTION	Actin and myosin fibres within the muscle slide together to create a pulling force.
ELASTIC RECOIL	The muscle membranes spring back (recoil) as the muscle is stretched.
MUSCLE REFLEXES	Rapid stretching causes the muscle to tighten to try to protect itself.

SPEED TRAINING PRINCIPLES

Plyometric exercise is intense, and so proper technique and adequate recovery is vital. Muscle aching is likely to be greater than for general bodytoning and so recovery periods of up to three days may be required. Initially plyometric training sessions may be practised once a week as a single component of a wider training programme. Even for experienced trainers plyometrics need not be practised more than twice a week and not on two consecutive days. In addition, plyometrics should not be practised all year round, but in specific periods (see p. 102) when speed training is emphasised.

Before practising plyometric drills, users must have a good basic level of fitness and a firm foundation of strength training. This strength training must have progressed from machines to free weights and you should have used some of the specialist lift movements, most importantly, the squat and dead lift actions. You should have no injuries at present, and be within the recommended weight and body fat range for your body type. Make sure that you are wearing supportive footwear which enables you to jump and land safely.

BALANCE AND STABILITY TESTS

Before progressing to plyometric training, you must be able to perform the tests described in Table 18.2. If you are unable to perform these tests your balance and leg/ankle stability is not yet ready for plyometrics. Use test one as an exercise for one week and then use both test one and two for a further week. Once you can perform both tests well, you are ready to begin plyometrics.

Table 18.2 Balance and stability tests prior to performing plyometrics	
Stand on one leg and fold your arms. Hold the position without toppling over and using the other leg for a minimum of 20-30 seconds on each leg. Rest, and then stand on one leg again and fold your arms. Close your eyes and stay on one leg without toppling over or touching the other leg down for 5-10 seconds. Perform the exercise on each leg.	Place your feet hip width apart and jump on both feet, bending your ankles, knees and hips as you land and keeping your trunk relatively upright (maximum lean forwards of 30-40°). Perform the jump 5 times and then jump and twist to the right by 45°. Land and get your balance before jumping again and twisting to the left. Perform this action 3 times to each side without toppling. Your landing should be soft and controlled, keeping your body upright.

SQUAT JUMP

Goal To develop leg muscle speed and power.

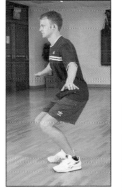

Technique Stand with your feet shoulder width apart, arms out to your sides at a 45° angle for balance. Bend your knees and angle forwards slightly from the waist into a squat position and then rapidly jump upwards as high as you can. As you land, sink down into the squat movement and repeat the jump again immediately without a pause.

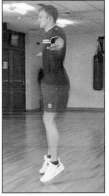

Points to note The landing for this action must be soft and absorbent. You should not hear or feel your feet stamp on the ground.

JUMP AND REACH

Goal To develop leg and arm power and speed.

Technique Stand with your feet shoulder width apart, arms out to your sides at a 45° angle for balance. Bend your knees and angle forwards slightly from the waist into a squat position and then rapidly jump upwards as high as you can, reaching overhead. As you land, sink down into the squat movement once more and repeat the action immediately without a pause.

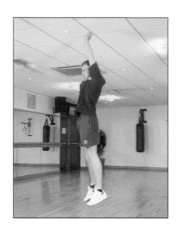

Points to note This action provides a rapid movement (flexion abduction) of the shoulder. If you suffer from clicking or painful shoulders it may not be suitable for you.

LUNGE JUMP

Goal To build power and speed in the leg muscles, emphasising single leg balance.

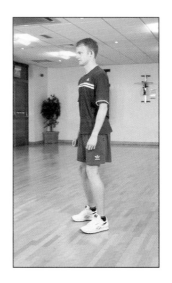

Technique Begin the movement standing with your feet just wider than shoulder width apart, arms angled out from your body by 45° for balance. Step forwards and practise the lunge action, ensuring that your knee passes over your foot and you do not go into a knock knee or bow leg position. Perform the lunge off each leg, keeping the step distance short (0.5–0.75m) and then build the speed up until you are jumping into the lunge position.

Points to note Make sure that you lower yourself into the lunge rather than falling into it. The speed of jumping upwards out of the lunge position should be greater than that of moving down.

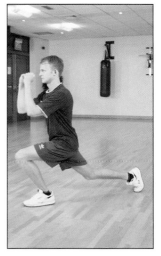

REPEATED HURDLE JUMP

Goal To build leg power and general agility.

Technique Set out a row of low objects to jump over (sticks, bands, etc.). These should be light enough to move easily if you knock into them. Stand in front of the first with your feet just wider than shoulder width apart, arms angled out from your body by 45° for balance. Jump over the first object, landing lightly, sink down and immediately jump over the second. Repeat this action for the whole row and then walk or gently jog back to the start. Perform three to five sets of this sequence and then rest to recover.

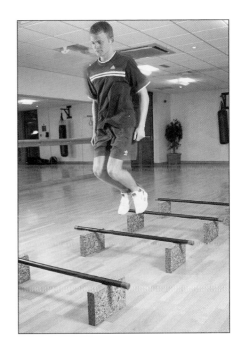

Points to note Strict form and concentration is vital on this movement. If your footwork begins to erode you will steadily get worse until you hit the last object. As soon as your technique begins to suffer, pause and then restart when your balance and alignment have been regained.

SINGLE LEG HOP

Goal To use a single leg action to build leg power.

Technique Stand on one leg and begin by hopping on the spot. Make sure that you sink through your ankle and knee and keep your upper body fairly upright. Once you can hop comfortably in one place, progress to repeated hopping forwards for five to ten steps and then walk back to the starting point to begin again.

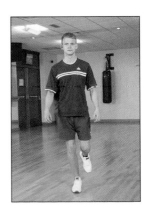

Points to note This exercise can be made harder by placing bands or low barriers on the ground and hopping over them to increase the jump height of each movement. Make sure that you remain balanced throughout the action. If your balance begins to degrade, stop and rest before you begin again.

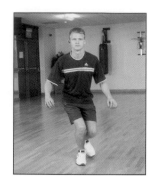

LATERAL JUMP

Goal To build leg power and develop side to side (lateral) leg stability.

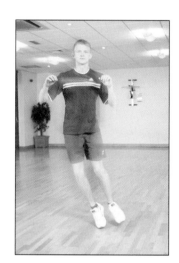

Technique Begin standing with your feet shoulder width apart, arms angled out from your body by 45° for balance. Jump sideways with both feet at the same time, sinking through your ankles and knees as you land. Perform the movement for 5 reps to the right, followed by 5 reps to the left. Rest and repeat the action.

Points to note As your feet touch the ground they stop moving, but your upper body motion continues. The result is a sliding or shearing stress on your knees and ankles. Practising this exercise will build up the muscle action which helps to resist these shearing forces.

PUNCH BAG PUSH

Goal To build power and speed in the chest, shoulders and arms.

Technique Begin facing a heavy punch bag with your arms shoulder width apart and bent. Straighten your arms to push the

18

BODYTONING

bag forwards and swing it away from you. As the bag swings back, receive it with your arms straight and bend your arms to absorb the bag's momentum. Take the bag all the way onto your chest and repeat the movement.

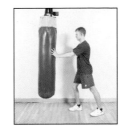

Points to note As the bag touches your hands on its back swing, your arms should be straight, but not locked out rigidly. By softening your arms slightly you will reduce shock on your wrists and elbows.

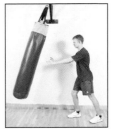

PUNCH BAG SIDE BEND

Goal To build speed and power in the trunk side flexors (oblique abdominals and quadratus lumborum).

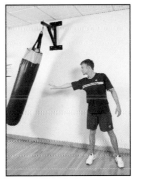

Technique Begin standing right side on to a punch bag with your feet astride and right arm out to the horizontal. Side bend and push the bag to the right with your straight arm. Allow the bag to swing away from you and, as it swings back, take its weight through your straight arm and side bend away from the bag to absorb its motion. Repeat the action to the left side.

Points to note It is important that the power for movement of the punch bag comes from trunk side bending rather than arm pushing. The arm must be kept straight throughout the movement.

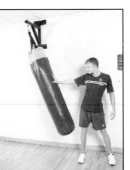
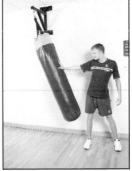

ROTARY TORSO PASS WITH PARTNER

Goal To build power and speed in the trunk rotator muscles (oblique abdominals).

Technique Stand with your feet astride, holding a medicine ball in both hands, with your elbows held into your sides. Your training partner should stand to your left side. Twist your trunk to your left and throw the medicine ball to your partner. Stay in the twisted position as your partner throws the ball back and 'unwind' your trunk as you catch the ball, twisting to the right. Twist back to the left and repeat. Repeat the action with your partner standing on your right side, throwing the ball to the right.

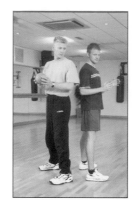

Points to note It is important that the power for movement of the medicine ball comes from trunk twisting rather than arm pushing. Keep your arms bent and elbows tucked into your sides throughout the movement.

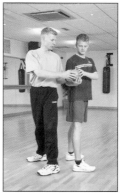

PARTIAL TRUNK CURL THROW

Goal To build power and speed in your trunk flexion muscles (rectus abdominis).

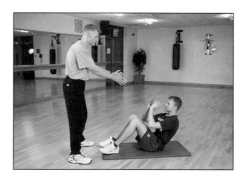

Technique Sit on a mat with your knees bent, with your training partner standing in front of you. Curl up, and ask your partner to throw a medicine ball towards your chest. Catch the ball with both hands and sink back to a partial trunk curl position, touching your lower back on the mat but keeping your shoulders off it. Sit forwards again, throwing the medicine ball to your partner.

Points to note Try to throw the medicine ball using trunk strength as well as arm strength. Only straighten your arms at the end of the movement as you sit forwards.

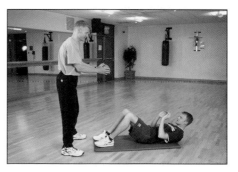

BODYTONING PROGRAMMES ‹

Bodytoning can be used for general fitness and also for specific toning of target areas. In addition, following injury it can be used to help regain lost function of a body part. In this chapter we will look at some examples of programmes for specific problems and the training modifications which may be needed for these. Remember that if you are training following an injury you should seek the advice of a qualified physiotherapist, and may find it helpful to train under the supervision of an experienced personal trainer.

BODYTONING AFTER PREGNANCY

The body undergoes major changes during pregnancy and it takes time to bring itself back to its pre-pregnancy condition. Changes in the joints of the pelvis, and hormones released in the run-up to childbirth make back pain a common occurrence after pregnancy. This situation is not helped by the new stresses and strains imposed on the body by lifting a newborn in activities such as bathing, transferring to a cot and using car seats.

The aim of bodytoning after pregnancy is to restrengthen the supporting muscles of the trunk and spine and to protect the body against injury as it recovers from the changes brought about by pregnancy.

Begin your programme with some core stability work and general cardiovascular (CV) exercise. Choose exercises which do not load the spine. For example, rather than using a squat exercise, we would choose a leg extension movement for leg muscle tone, as this exercise does not involve holding a weight. As you gain strength, practise some exercises to strengthen your back correctly for lifting. The hip hinge movement and lunge are especially useful for this. The former will teach you to bend correctly keeping your back straight and bending your knees. The latter will help to strengthen the leg muscles which provide the power for you to lift.

If you find you do not have enough time to go to a gym as often as you would like, use some band exercises in your workout which you can practise at home to maintain some of your muscle tone between visits to the gym.

Cross trainer 5–10 minutes

Seated machine chest press

Lat pull down

Abdominal hollowing (lying with knees bent)

Stability ball

Bands for legs

Hip hinge (hands on table)

BODYTONING FOR A STRONG BACK

Backpain affects four out of five people at some time in their lives. One of the major risk factors for back pain is repeated bending actions and poor lifting on top of a back which is weak and stiff through a sedentary lifestyle. Bodytoning can address this problem on a number of fronts. It can help to teach you the correct methods of bending and lifting, improve your alignment and strengthen both the muscles which support your spine and the muscles which provide the power for lifting. Regular bodytoning exercise will not make you immune to back pain, but it will make it considerably less likely. And, if back pain should strike, a fit toned body is more able to cope, so your recovery is likely to be quicker and more complete.

Begin with core stability training, first on a mat and then with some work on a gym ball. As this progresses, put in some leg strengthening activities coupled with lifting techniques. The most important movements here are the dumb-bell lunge and the hip hinge action, followed eventually by the good morning action. Lifting techniques are addressed with the dead lift and modifications of this movement. The back muscles themselves are worked with the spinal extension movement, building up the endurance or 'muscle holding time' of this exercise.

CV work – cross trainer, cycle (upright sitting), brisk treadmill walk (not run)
Lat pull down
Seated rowing (machine)
Heel slide
Bent knee fall out
Gymball
Hyperextension 10s hold (weeks 2–4) progressing to 30s hold (weeks 4–6)
Hip hinge (weeks 2–4) progressing to good morning (weeks 4–6)
Squat
Dead lift (from bench initially)

BODYTONING FOR A FLAT STOMACH

There are several factors which go together to produce a lax stomach. Poor tone of the abdominal muscles and lengthening of these muscles are major factors, as is body weight. All of these factors must be addressed to create a flat stomach.

Bodytoning must be used first to pull the abdominal muscles in. For this we use a *hollowing* action initially in standing and then lying on the back (p. 69). Once this has been achieved, build up the holding time of these movements to keep the abdominal muscles tighter for a longer period. The next stage is to *shorten* the abdominal muscles by pulling the two ends of the central muscle (rectus abdominis) together maximally. Now we use a modified trunk curl movement, tilting the pelvis to target the lower abdominals and curling the trunk to work the upper abs. Finally, we increase the variety of movements by working on the trunk rotators. This type of workout will involve quite a few abdominal movements and so staggered sets are used, placing one ab exercise between sets on other body parts. In addition, to get the final results that we are hoping for the intensity of work must be increased by using eccentric training and peak contractions.

Weeks 1–3

General warm-up cycle 5 min

Abdominal hollowing in standing

Chest press

Heel slide

Lat pull down

Bent knee fall out

Lunge

Weeks 3–5

Rowing machine 10 min

Bent knee fall out

Shoulder press

Rotary torso machine

Squat

Abdominal machine (normal weeks 3–4, peak contraction weeks 4–5)

Cross trainer

Dumb-bell sidebend

BODYTONING FOR A FIRM BUM

The bum muscles are the gluteals (Fig. 12.1(a)). The gluteus maximus is the major muscle forming most of the bum, while the gluteus medius is at the side, helping to create the hollow at the side of the upper hip. The muscles are immensely strong and require quite hard work. However, in some cases they may not be working at all!

In many individuals, especially those who have had back pain in the past, the gluteal muscles are in very poor condition. This means that people have problems bending correctly and tend to bend only from the back rather than from the hips. One of the results of this is that the hamstring muscles (which also work on the hip) become very tight and thick and the gluteals are flat and lax. To redress this imbalance we have to get the gluteals working correctly, and only when this has been achieved can we move on to actually working them hard.

Here is a simple test of the state of your gluteal muscles. Lie on the floor and bend one leg at the knee. Now, keeping the knee bent, try to lift the whole leg up as high as you can. When you do this, your bum should get so tight that the muscles feel toned and hard. If they feel weak and wobbly, the chances are that your gluteal muscles are not working correctly.

We begin with gluteal isolation exercises. First, lie on the floor on your back and simply squeeze your buttocks together. Tighten and hold them tight, building up to a count of ten. When you can do this, bend your knees up and try to form a shoulder bridge. Here, you lift your hips, tightening your gluteals as you do so, until your knees, hips and shoulders are in a straight line. Hold this position for a count of five and then lower. Once you can perform this exercise, tightening your gluteals five times, holding each rep for a count of five, you can begin the programme shown.

Cross trainer – 5 min forwards, 5 min backwards

Gymball single leg bridge

Lunge

Shoulder press with bodybar

Glut toner (prone hip extension unit)

Squat

Seated rowing

Active hamstring stretch (p. 74)

BODYTONING FOR WEIGHT LOSS

In order to lose weight basically you need to use more energy in the form of exercise or general activity than you are taking in as food – this creates what is known as a *negative energy balance* – and you need to use some of the energy you are storing as fat. Exercise which increases your heart rate and breathing rate for a prolonged period will effectively burn off fat, but it must be linked to a reduction in high energy foods. These are typically fatty and sugary foods, especially convenience foods such as biscuits, crisps, fried foods, alcohol and sweets. Try to reduce your intake of these foods and increase the amount of exercise designed to raise your heart rate, so-called cardiovascular or CV exercises. In addition when people are overweight (or really overfat) they usually also have poor muscle tone and 'flabby' lax muscles. Muscle toning exercises should also therefore be included. One of the best ways to achieve results in this area is to use circuit weight training. This type of activity uses very light weights and high numbers of repetitions, and alternates body parts. You would therefore work arms–legs–trunk and repeat this sequence throughout the session.

Cross trainer 5–10 min
Seated chest press 30 sec
Bench squat (powerbar) 30 sec
Trunk curl 30 sec

Cycle 5 min
Lat pull down 30 sec
Thigh abductor 30 sec
Rotary torso 30 sec
Rowing machine 5 min

Dumb-bell lateral raise 30 sec

Lunge (no weight) 30 sec

Pelvic lift 30 sec

BODYTONING TO BUILD MUSCLE

To build muscle tissue we need to work harder than we would do in everyday life (p. 62). This extra work challenges our muscles so much that it actually causes microscopic damage. This so-called micro-damage is not a negative thing, however. Indeed it causes the muscle to grow stronger in an attempt to be more able to cope with future demands. In order to grow stronger the muscle must have an available supply of nutrients from food, and more importantly adequate rest to allow it to regrow. These are the ingredients for building muscle then: intense training, good diet and plenty of rest, including daytime 'power naps', to allow the muscle time to build.

We use multijoint exercises initially, those which work three or four muscles at the same time, such as the bench press. Once we have been training for some time and the exercises start to feel easy, we can use some of the advanced training techniques given in chapter 10.

Warm-up cross trainer or rower 5–10 min

Bench press 12/10/8 reps

Seated rowing 10/8

Shoulder press 12/10/8

Lat pull down 10/8

Squat 12/10/8

Lunge 10/8

Calf raise 15/12

Trunk curl 20/20

Dips 12/10

Triceps extension 12/10 (superset)

Chin 12/10

Arm curl 12/10 (superset)

BODYTONING FOR POSTURE

To effectively correct posture we really need to identify our particular postural type and use exercises tailored to this (p. 41). However, there are some general guidelines for overall postural exercise programmes. There are two areas that need to be addressed with postural exercise. The first is the area of the pelvis and tummy (*pelvic girdle*) and the second the area of the shoulders and upper spine (*thoracic girdle*).

We use core stability training to flatten the tummy and improve the support to the lower back. This allows us to pull the tummy in firmly and provides the body's central foundation for posture. The equivalent action in the upper body is to draw the shoulder blades in and slightly down and to lengthen the spine. Several exercises help with this action, including rowing actions and spinal extension movements.

With postural re-education strength is a secondary concern. The primary aim is to tone muscle and improve *postural holding*. This is the ability of a muscle to tighten and hold you in correct alignment over a period of time. For this we use light resistances but hold the muscle contraction for 10–30 seconds. Postural exercises often form part of a total workout. Choose some of the movements below to add a postural dimension to your training.

Heel slide

Gymball various (eg supine back stretch)

Dumb-bell rowing

Shoulder retraction machine

Hyperextension and hold

Scapular stabilisation using band (p. 169)

BODYTONING FOR BREATHING COMPLAINTS

There are many breathing (respiratory) problems which benefit from exercise. Asthma in children and young adults, and bronchitis in seniors are just two of the many chest problems to benefit from regular exercise. Exercise will achieve two major things. First, the efficiency of the lungs is improved. The way the lungs pull in air and how the oxygen from this air travels in the blood to the working muscle can both improve with exercise. Second, with many chest conditions, the way the ribs work alters and the chest becomes either very flat or barrel shaped and inflexible. This has a knock-on effect on the area of the spine between the shoulder blades (thoracic spine). Specific bodytoning exercises can improve chest expansion and work on the thoracic spine to help alleviate pain.

For exercises targeted at specific respiratory conditions you should consult a qualified physiotherapist. However, here are some exercises which will help to expand the chest and improve breathing in general.

CV work (cycle, rower, or cross trainer) beginning with low intensity (60% maximum heart rate) for 3–7 minutes. Extend time to 8–12 minutes over a period of 10 days and then increase intensity to 70% HRmax.

Dumb-bell pull over (light weight)

Seated chest press

'Pec deck' (seated arm adduction)

Seated pulley row

Rotary torso

Shoulder bracing

Thoracic stretch on gymball

BODYTONING FOR CIRCULATION PROBLEMS

There are a number of circulatory problems which limit a person's ability to walk or jog. Often the limiting factor is aching and pain which comes on after a certain distance is walked. Exercise can improve walking ability and the amount of activity which can be performed before the legs become too tired (exercise tolerance). In addition the blood flow through the leg muscles and general leg muscle tone can be improved.

CV exercises should be practised to the point at which leg pain just begins to appear. With time, it will take longer for the pain to occur (exercise tolerance has improved) and fitness will increase.

Cycle/recumbent cycle/cross trainer – low intensity (40% maximum heart rate) work up to pain onset.

Dumb-bell shoulder raise (1–2 kg)
Trunk rotation

Repeat CV exercise to pain onset
Stretching

BODYTONING FOR HEART PROBLEMS

Many years ago patients were told to go home and rest after they had experienced a heart attack or had heart (cardiac) surgery. Nowadays things have changed and a closely monitored programme of cardiac rehabilitation is normally recommended under the supervision of a qualified physiotherapist. However, there are things that you can do to help yourself. All exercise must be pulse monitored, that is, you must wear a commercially available heart rate monitor. You should aim to keep your pulse rate in a training zone dictated by your age (see p. 20). Generally begin by training at 30–40 per cent of your maximal age-related heart rate and work continually for 15–20 minutes. Build this intensity and duration up to 50–60 per cent of maximum heart rate for 20–30 minutes per session. Practise three or four sessions per week. If your heart rate goes above your target, slow down gradually rather than stopping. If it goes below your target, gradually increase the intensity to bring it back up again. Each workout should begin with a warm-up designed to increase your heart rate to the training zone over a period of 3–5 minutes, and end with an equivalent cool-down. Your twenty minutes exercise can either be performed on a single piece of CV equipment or as a light circuit using several pieces of apparatus.

After heart surgery the chest and shoulders tend to be very stiff and so light stretching is recommended. Some exercises such as the shoulder press and lat pull down offer a good stretch simply because they involve overhead reaching actions, so these are particularly useful.

Either: 20 min CV (recumbent cycle, static cycle, cross trainer, walking on treadmill).
Or: 5 min uphill walk on treadmill

Seated shoulder press	10 reps
Seated leg press	10
Trunk rotation	5 each side
Lat pull down	10
Seated rowing	10
Side bend	5 each side

BODYTONING FOR ACHES AND PAINS

After you have had an injury, bodytoning can be used to build the area up again, remove stiffness and generally increase your confidence in a region. You can of course use general exercise for the rest of your body and need only use the specific exercise therapy for the area of your body which has been injured. For example, if you have had an ankle injury you can still use a seated bench press for your upper body and a rotary torso machine for your trunk. The injury only limits lower body movements and so the specific movements given below must be built into your general workout. The programmes featured are 'add-ons' or 'substitutions' to your general workout.

Frozen shoulder

A frozen shoulder occurs when the bag surrounding the ball and socket joint of the shoulder (*the joint capsule*) becomes stiff and thickened. This limits movements, especially twisting and reaching overhead, and also gives muscle weakness. In parallel with a course of physiotherapy, shoulder stretching and strengthening can help. The outward twisting (*lateral rotation*) movements of the arm are limited so these should be addressed. Overhead reaching will be very painful so these are best left to the physiotherapist, but reaching forwards is normally less painful.

CV work with cycle – avoid rower or cross trainer

Seated chest press (narrow grip)
Lateral rotation with dumb-bell (light weight, aiming for full range motion)

Seated row machine
Normal leg and trunk work

Tennis elbow

Tennis elbow is an inflammation and scarring of the point of attachment of the forearm straightening muscles (extensors) to the bone of the elbow. It causes pain when lifting anything with the knuckles downwards and pain when gripping tightly on small narrow objects. Both of these movements should be avoided. There is often an involvement with the nerves which run from the neck through the elbow to the hand, and your physiotherapist will check this out.

The aim of bodytoning exercise is to work the forearm muscles lightly to stimulate regrowth of healthy tissue in the affected area. To do this exercise must be practised just below the point that pain occurs. Do not just work the elbow thinking that you can 'work the pain off'. This will increase swelling and make the condition last much longer.

The key exercises are wrist extension, the reverse curl and forearm twisting (pronation and supination). Each should be performed with a light weight, even just a stick to begin with. With time you will find you can perform more exercise before the pain comes on.

CV work avoiding gripping activities (cycle leaning on the handlebars but not gripping, cross trainer legs only, treadmill)

Wrist extension
Reverse curl
Forearm twisting (stick and then hammer bell)

Normal leg and trunk exercises

Hip replacement

Hip replacements are among the most successful bone and joint (orthopaedic) operations. Bodytoning is helpful afterwards to build up muscle around the hips and waist and to reduce the chances of limping. This often occurs as a result of the pain experienced in the months prior to the operation and continues as a habit after surgery.

Two movements to avoid after a hip operation are crossing the legs (forced adduction) and taking the knee upwards towards the chest (hip flexion beyond 90°). In addition jarring stresses on the hip should be limited (jogging on hard surfaces).

Bodytoning aims to strengthen the gluteal muscles (hip extension) and the muscles at the side of the hip and pelvis (hip hitching action). Normal CV and upper body work can be used, tailored to your current fitness level.

CV work (recumbent cycle, static cycle)
Bridging on a mat, building to bridging on gym ball
Leg extension
Hip abduction seated (limited range)
Hip adductor on a multihip unit (to centre of body only)

Normal upper body work

Knee ligament injuries

The most common knee ligament injury is to the ligament on the inside of the knee, called the *medial collateral ligament* or MCL. This is typically injured when you press your knee inwards as the foot is on the ground and your body weight is taken through your leg. This movement forces the knee joint to open slightly on the inside and overstretches the ligament. After this type of injury the thigh muscles (*quadriceps*) often become very weak and the knee is stiff and unable to bend properly. Bodytoning aims to address these two factors, strengthening the quads and encouraging knee bending actions.

Initially quadriceps activities such as the leg extension movement are used because they are non-weight-bearing, that is to say, you are not putting your body weight through your foot. Non-weight-bearing actions are less painful after this type of injury and so are used first. As the joint improves you can use partial weight-bearing movements (taking some weight through the knee), such as leg press, and finally full weight-bearing exercise, where you take your whole weight through the knee, such as lunges and squats.

CV work encouraging knee bending (cycle, rower – leave the foot free with straps loose to allow the shin bones to twist rather than the knee)

Leg extension (limited range of motion)
Leg curl (encouraging knee bending)
Hip abductor machine

Normal upper body and trunk exercise

Hamstring pulls

The hamstring muscles at the back of the thigh are commonly pulled by sudden mistimed movements. Sudden lunging or a rapid unprepared sprint can cause the muscle to tear. Injury usually occurs either to the fleshy central part of the muscle (*mid belly tear*) or at the end of the muscle at the point where it attaches to the sitting bone (*ischial origin*). The aim of bodytoning is to regain the strength which will have been lost following injury and to rebuild flexibility. In addition, once these two aims have been achieved the speed and power of the muscle must be redeveloped as the hamstrings more than any other muscle work for rapid power movements in sport.

Early development of strength focuses on broadening the muscle to break the muscle fibres free of clotted swelling deep inside the muscle. Broadening of this type can be achieved with a leg curl action. Stretching using active knee extension (AKE – p. 74) aims to lengthen the muscle under control. Once the muscle pain begins to reduce, actions which involve movement over the hip and knee combined are vital. Lunges and squats are useful now, and these can gradually build in terms of speed to controlled plyometrics including jump squat and jump lunges, followed eventually by hopping actions.

CV work within painless range-cycle, cross trainer, stair climber

Leg curl – early stage only

Hamstring stretching

Lunge

Squat

Plyometrics – dumb-bell jumping squat, jumping lunge

Normal upper body and trunk exercise

Sprained ankle

An ankle sprain is a common problem, but because it is so common this injury is often taken far too lightly. In fact, wrongly treated, ankle sprains can leave a person with a permanent limp, giving problems in the whole leg in later life. The two factors of importance following an ankle sprain are strength of the ankle muscles to support the body weight and stop the ankle giving way, and flexibility to allow normal walking. When you stand on one leg in bare feet you will notice your ankle and shin muscles flickering as they contract rapidly to support (*stabilise*) your ankle. This is an indication of how important these muscles are to the stability of the ankle and stopping it giving way and twisting again. All of the shin muscles are important to this function but those on the outside of the shin (*the peronei muscles*) are especially needed. In addition to specific ankle exercises, such as heel raises, single leg standing movements initially performed slowly (lunging) and then more rapidly (hopping) are vital. These can progress to side to side movements such as lateral jumps in plyometrics (p. 194). The movement of the ankle which is normally limited is *dorsiflexion*, which occurs when you take your knee forwards over your foot, and *inversion*, where the sole of your foot swings inwards. A squat movement or working on a stair climber will work dorsiflexion, providing you keep your foot flat on the pedal and do not rise up onto your toes.

> CV work – cross trainer (keep foot flat)
> Squat
> Lunge
> Heel raise – standing
> Heel raise – seated
>
> Plyometrics (when strength built up) – squat jump, hopping, lateral jumps
>
> Normal upper body and trunk work

Torn calf muscle

There are two calf muscles, the gastrocnemius is the larger of the two and lies on the surface (superficial) while the soleus is deeper and smaller. The gastrocnemius works to propel the body forwards, as in running and jumping for example, and so is easily torn in sport. The soleus works to sway your body forwards and back in a standing posture, to maintain balance.

Following a calf tear the muscle must be built up again and its flexibility improved. Heel raises will strengthen the calf: seated heel raises targeting the soleus and standing calf raises the gastrocnemius. Both exercises will also stretch the calf providing the heel is allowed to drop right down. In addition the calf may be stretched separately by facing a wall, keeping the feet flat and leaning forwards (p. 76).

Once strength and flexibility have been regained, speed and power should be worked with plyometrics. Jumping, hopping and bounding will all work the calf to gradually increasing intensities.

CV work – cycle, recumbent (weeks 1–2), rower, cross trainer (weeks 3–4), treadmill walk (weeks 2–4), treadmill jog (weeks 3–6)

Calf raise – seated and standing (weeks 1–4)

Stretching

Squat

Lunge

Jumping dumb-bell squat (weeks 4–6)

Low hopping (weeks 4–6)

Hopping over bar (weeks 6–8)

Treadmill run on incline, and flat sprint (weeks 6–8)

Pain between the shoulder blades

Pain between the shoulder blades can come from several causes, two of the most common being stiffness and stress on the thoracic spine due to a round shoulder posture and muscle weakness or spasm in the shoulder bracing (retractor) muscles which run between the shoulder blades. Bodytoning in conjunction with physiotherapy can help both problems.

Shoulder bracing movements such as seated rowing and single arm dumb-bell rows are used, and thoracic flexibility movements such as side bends and spinal stretching over a gymball are also helpful.

CV work paying attention to alignment – any

Seated row

Single arm dumb-bell row

Spinal extension hold

Spinal stretch over gymball

Lat pull down

Lateral dumb-bell raise

Normal leg work

acclimatisation The body getting used to an environment

accommodating resistance Resistance changes as you move

acetylcholine A nerve conductor

actin Part of the muscle protein responsible for muscle action

adenine A chemical found in energy products within the body

adenine diphosphate (ADP) Molecule left when ATP has given up some of its energy

adenosine triphosphate (ATP) A large molecule capable of storing energy

aerobic Producing energy with oxygen

alarm reaction A body response which results from a challenge

alveolus The air sack within the lung

amino acid Part of a protein or body building food unit

antagonist A muscle on the opposite side of the joint to the prime mover

assistant mover The muscle which helps the prime mover

assisted movement A movement which is helped by a machine

barbell A long bar with a weight at either end, generally used with both hands

basal metabolic rate Tickover rate of your body at rest

biarticular A muscle which travels over two joints

biceps Your arm bending muscles

blood pressure The pressure the blood exerts due to the pumping of the heart

body fat The fat beneath the skin and around organs

bucket handle Movement of chest where the movement goes out sideways

burn The pain during muscle contraction

centre of gravity The balance point of an object

contraction Muscle pulling to create force

deltoid Your shoulder cap muscles

developmental stretching Stretches designed to increase your flexibility

diaphragm Sheet of muscle beneath the chest

diastolic The part of the blood pressure due to heart relaxation

disaccharide A simple energy sugar

dislocation A joint coming out of its socket

DOMS (Delayed Onset Muscle Soreness) The pain felt one or two days following an intense workout

dumb-bell A short bar with two weights used in one hand

duration The length of time you spend exercising

effort The force created to lift the weights

elastic recoil The energy a muscle produces as it relaxes under tension

electrolyte A charged particle within the body

enzymes Substances which help to create chemical reactions within your body

exercised Carrying out any activity (contract to training)

exhaustion phase The body failing to cope with a challenge

extensor A muscle which straightens a joint

facet joint Two small joints lying on either side of each spinal unit (vertebrae)

fasiculus A bundle of muscle fibres

fast twitch A muscle fibre built for power

flexor A muscle which bends a joint

force–velocity trade-off Faster movements giving less force

frequency The number of times you perform an exercise

gastrocnemius The long and superficial calf muscle

glucose A sugar within the blood

gluteals Your bottom muscles

gluteus maximus Your large bottom muscle

gluteus medius Your large bottom/hip muscle

glycaemic index A measure of the energy producing capacity of food

glycogen A partially digested sugar in the blood or muscle

glycolysis Producing energy in the body without oxygen

group action A number of muscles working together

haemoglobin The oxygen-carrying substance within the blood

hamstring Your knee-bending muscle

heartbeat The pumping of the heart, average values are 60–70 beats per minute (BPM)

hip abductor The muscle which pulls your legs apart

hip adductor The muscle which pulls your legs together

hip flexor Your hip bending muscle

hypertrophy Building a muscle

iliopsoas Your deep hip muscle

impingement Trapping something as a joint moves

imprinting spine Gently pressing the small of your back against a mat

intensity How hard an exercise is

internal oblique The sheet-like muscles standing on top of the transversus abdominis

ischaemia The blood flow through a muscle being restricted

knurlings The hatchings on a bar

lactate accumulation curve A measure of the build-up of lactic acid in the body

lactate threshold The point at which the body begins to produce lactic acid

lactic acid A poison produced within the muscle which causes aching

latissimus dorsi The muscle at the side of your chest beneath your arm

lean body mass Your body with the fat stripped off

length–tension relationship The relationship between the length of the muscle and the power it can create

local blood flow The flow of blood through the local muscle area

lordotic posture An increased curvature in the base of the spine

lumbar lordosis The curve in the lower spine

lumbar spine Lower spine

maintenance stretching Stretches designed to maintain your current level of flexibility

mass Another term for the weight of an object

metabolism The energy producing actions of your body

mobility Exercises to increase your range of motion, another word for stretching

monosaccharide A simple energy sugar

motor nerve A nerve carrying impulses for movement

motor unit A small nerve and the muscle fibres it supplies

movement muscle A muscle which contracts to create a movement

multifidus A small muscle lying between the bones of the spine

musculo-tendinous junction The joining part between the muscle and tendon

myelin sheath The insulating sheath around a nerve

myofibrils A number of muscle fibres joined together

myogenic Changes within muscle chemicals

myosin Part of the muscle protein responsible for muscle action

neurogenic Changes within muscle nerves

neuromuscular junction The joint between the joint and muscle

neutral position The optimal alignment of the pelvis and lower spine

neutralisers A muscle which stops an unwanted movement of a joint

non-contractile tissue Tissues which do not contract, such as ligaments and tendons

nutrients Vital products extracted by your body from foods

OBLA Onset of Blood Lactate Accumulation, a measure of the endurance capacity of a muscle

oblique abdominals Sheet like muscles which surround your trunk

olympic bar A competitive bar used for weight lifting

optimal posture The theoretical perfect posture

overload An exercise which challenges the body

oxidation Breaking foodstuffs down in the presence of oxygen

parallel Muscle fibres running in the same line

pectorals Your large chest muscles

pelvic floor The muscles between your legs

pennate Muscle fibres fanning out

peronei The muscles which swing your foot outwards

phosphates The energy unit of the body

phosphocreatine (PC) The immediate energy store of the body

plateauing Reaching a sticking point within a movement

polysaccharide A complex energy sugar

preferential hypertrophy Building some muscle fibres within a large muscle but not others

prime mover The muscle which carries out a movement

progressing Gradually making exercises harder

pronation Twisting the forearm downwards

pulse raising An exercise which increases the heart rate or pulse rate and makes you breathe deeply

pump The pain and puffiness of a muscle after exercise

pump handle Movement of the lungs where the breast bone goes up and forwards

quadriceps Your knee straightening muscles

reciprocal innervation The process by which one muscle contracts as the opposing muscle relaxes

recruited Nervous impulses causing a muscle to contract

rectus femoris The kicking muscle in the thigh

rehearsal Practising the technique involved in a particular exercise before any weight is used

relaxin hormone A hormone which affects the joints of the pelvis during pregnancy and childbirth

resistance How difficult it is to lift a weight, or stretch a band

resistance phase The body trying to cope with a challenge

ribose Part of the energy foods in the body

rotator cuff Your shoulder twisting muscles

sarcolemna One of the membranes of the muscles

sarcomere The basic muscle unit

saturated fat A type of fat which comes from animals

shoulder retractors The muscles which pull your shoulders back

slow twitch A muscle fibre built for endurance

soleus The deeper and shorter calf muscle

somatotype Your body type

spasm A muscle being permanently contracted

spinal disc The cushion between two spinal bones

spinal extensors Your back muscles

stabilisers Muscle which holds a joint together

steady state Producing the same amount of energy as you use up

super compensation Muscles changing as a result of training

supporting base The base of an object which lies on the floor

systolic The part of the blood pressure due to heart contraction

task muscle A muscle which contracts to create a movement

thorocolumbar fascia The tight area on your back and lower spine

tibialis anterior The muscle which pulls your foot upwards

tissue stiffness The resistance a tissue gives

trained An activity which caused the body to change (*see also* exercised)

transversus abdominis The deepest of the sheet-like muscles of the tummy

triceps Your arm straightening muscles

triglyceride A component of fat

tropomyosin A microscopic part of the muscle

troponin A microscopic part of the muscle

type The style of an exercise

umbilicus Your tummy button

unsaturated fat A type of fat which comes from plants

velocity How fast a movement is

visualisation Imagining the movements you are about to carry out

American College of Sports Medicine (1978) 'The Recommended Quantity and Quality of Exercise for Developing and Maintaining Fitness in Healthy Adults', *Medicine and Science in Sports and Exercise*, 10: vii–x.

—— (1990) 'The Recommended Quantity and Quality of Exercise for Developing and Maintaining Cardio Respiratory and Muscular Fitness in Healthy Adults', *Medicine and Science in Sports and Exercise*, 22: 265–74.

—— (2002) 'Progression Models in Resistance Training for Healthy Adults', *Medicine and Science in Sports and Exercise*, 34: 364–80.

Astrand, P.O. and Rodahl, K. (1986) *Textbook of Work Physiology*, McGraw-Hill, New York.

Bandy, W.D. and Irion, J.M. (1994) 'The effect of time on static stretch on the flexibility of the hamstring muscles', *Physical Therapy*, 74 (9): 845–52.

Barnard, R.J., Gardner, G.W., Diaco, N.V. and Kattus, A.A. (1973) 'Cardiovascular responses to sudden strenuous exercise: Heart rate, blood pressure, and ECG', *Journal of Applied Physiology*, 34: 883.

Bean, A. (1997) *The Complete Guide to Sports Nutrition* (3rd ed), A&C Black, London.

Below P.R., Mora-Rodriguez, R. and Gonzalez-Alonso, J. (1995) 'Fluid and Carbohydrate Ingestion Independently Improve Performance during 1 Hour of Intense Exercise', *Medicine and Science in Sport and Exercise*, 27: 200–10.

Brook, G.A. (1987) 'Amino Acid and Protein Metabolism during Exercise and Recovery', *Medicine and Science in Sport and Exercise*, 19: 150–6.

Cappozzo, A., Felici, F. and Figura, F. (1985) 'Lumbar Spine Loading during Half Squat Exercises', *Medicine and Science in Sports and Exercise*, 17(5): 613–20.

Fiatarone, M.E., Marks, E., Ryan, C. and Evans, W. (1990) 'High intensity strength training in nonagenarians: Effects on skeletal muscle', *Journal of the American Medical Association*, 263: 3029–34.

Gettman, L.R. and Pollock, M.L. (1981) 'Circuit weight training: A critical review of its physiological benefits', *The Physician and Sports Medicine*, 9(1): 44–60.

Hettinger, T.L and Muller, E.A. (1953) 'Muskelleistung and Muskeltraining', *International Journal of Physiology*, 15: 111.

Jette, A. and Branch, L. (1981) 'The Framingham disability study II: Physical disability among the aging', *American Journal of Public Health*, 71: 1211–16.

Leatt, P., Reilly, T. and Troup, J.G.D. (1986) 'Spinal Loading during Circuit Weight Training and Running', *British Journal of Sports Medicine*, 20(3): 119–24.

Mainwood, G. and Renaud, J. (1985) 'The Effect of Acid-Base on Fatigue of Skeletal Muscle', *Canadian Journal of Physiology and Pharmacology*, 63: 403–16.

Morganti, C., Nelson, M., Fiatarone, E., Crawford, B. and Evans, W. (1995) 'Strength improvements with one year of progressive resistance training in older women', *Medicine and Science in Sports and Exercise*, 27: 906–12.

Norris, C.M. (1999) *The Complete Guide to Stretching*, A&C Black, London.

—— (2001) *Abdominal Training: Enhancing Core Stability*, A&C Black, London.

Seyle, H. (1956) *The Stress of Life*, McGraw-Hill, New York.

Taylor, D.C., Dalton, J., Seaber, A.V. and Garrett W.E. (1990) 'The viscoelastic properties of muscle tendon units', *American Journal of Sports Medicine*, 18: 300–9.

Tyrrell, A.R., Reilly, T. and Troup, J.G.D. (1985) 'Circadian Variation in Stature and the Effects of Spinal Loading', *Spine*, 10: 161–4.

Waterman-Storer, C.M. (1991) 'The Cytoskeleton of Skeletal Muscle: Is it Affected by Exercise? A Brief Review', *Medicine and Science in Sports and Exercise*, 23: 1249–54.

Wilmore, J.H., Parr, R.B. and Girandola, R.N. (1978) 'Physiological alterations consequent to circuit weight training', *Medicine and Science in Sports and Exercise*, 10: 79–84.

INDEX